Menopause Without Medicine

*D*r. Linda Ojeda has written a book that should be read by any woman concerned with planning for the future . . . . MENOPAUSE WITHOUT MEDICINE could be described as a 'wellness bible.' It really gives women an overall picture of their bodies and how to keep [them] running to optimum proficiency. As menstruation is the beginning of a woman's reproductive cycle; menopause should be seen as the culmination, not the bitter ending." — *Whole Life Times*

*M*ENOPAUSE WITHOUT MEDICINE is more than another overview of symptoms: it probes the underlying beliefs and concepts about aging which can prove self-defeating, and presents suggestions and programs designed to combat and minimalize the depression and stress associated with menopause." — *The Midwest Book Review*

*E*xemplifying recent, more enlightened attitudes toward menopause, Ojeda regards her subject as a part of the natural evolution of a woman's body, not as a condition to treat or mask. She believes further that menopause is not the death of womanhood but the birth of a new life stage. Hence, she focuses on wellness, recommending natural ways—including dietary modifications, vitamins, exercise, and attitudinal adaptation—to cope with the body's changes during menopause . . . . She also packs the book with appendixes, charts, recipes, and suggested resources. These, combined with the accessible, reassuring, and *female* tone of her writing, make this a very useful resource." — *Booklist*

*A*n excellent book . . . . It is often easy to find books that tell us how wonderful estrogen is for menopausal women. It is not so easy to find a book that talks about alternatives. Linda Ojeda has written such a book." — Miriam Diamond, *Elizabeth Blackwell Health Center for Women*

A Selection of the Doubleday Health Bookclub

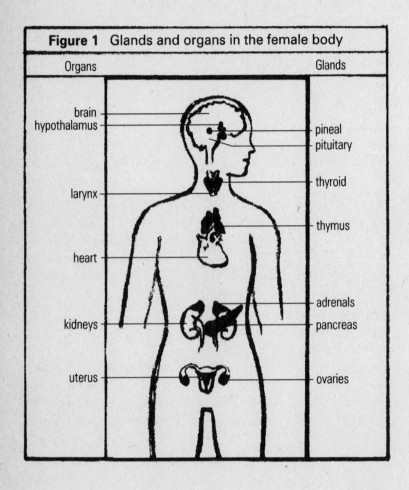

Figure 1 Glands and organs in the female body

Organs

Glands

brain
hypothalamus

pineal
pituitary

thyroid

larynx

thymus

heart

adrenals

kidneys

pancreas

uterus

ovaries

Menopause
Without
Medicine

Linda Ojeda, Ph.D.

Hunter
House

HUNTER HOUSE INC., PUBLISHERS
P.O. Box 2914
Alameda CA 94501-0914
ISBN 0-89793-178-5

Project Editor	*Production Manager*
LISA E. LEE	PAUL J. FRINDT
Copy Editors	*Book Design*
JACKIE MELVIN, MALI APPLE	DIAN-AZIZA OOKA
Proofreaders	*Cover Design*
JANIS PARIS, SUSAN BURKHARDT	JIL WEIL
Sales & Marketing	*Illustrations*
CORRINE M. SAHLI	DANIEL NYIRI
Publicity & Promotion	Scheduling & Administration
DARCY COHAN	MARÍA JESÚS AGUILÓ
Customer Support	*Order Fulfillment*
SHARON R.A. OLSON, SAM BREWER	A&A QUALITY SHIPPING SERVICES

Publisher
KIRAN S. RANA

✦

Set in Goudy, Journal, and Zurich by 847 Communications, Alameda CA

Manufactured in the United States of America

To my husband, Roland

✦

Contents

PART ONE
Menopause:
Symptoms and Remedies

PART TWO
Preparing for the Later Years

Antioxidants
B Vitamins
DHEA

PART THREE
Nutrition for Life:
A Woman's Guide

Protein
Carbohydrates
Fiber
Fat
Water

16   **Eliminate the Negative** 245
Nonfood Additives
Sugar
Salt
Caffeine
Alcohol
Cigarettes

17   **Putting Your Diet into Action** 257
Charting for Health
Are You Depriving Your Body of Nutrients?
Reading Your Body
Eating for Life

18   **Designing Your Supplement Program** 267

Appendix A: A Basic Nutrient Formula
    for Women 274

Appendix B: Clinical Symptoms of Nutrient
    Deficiencies 276

Appendix C: Major Nutrient Guide 279

Appendix D: Strengthening Exercises
    for Women 285

    Notes 302

    Glossary 317

    Resources 323

    Index 327

List of Illustrations

Throughout the text, the superscript numbers refer to the Notes, which are arranged by chapter.

Most common health and medical terms used in the text are further defined in the glossary.

Acknowlegments

Writing a book is not a solitary endeavor. Many creative people contribute to making the work more than a collection of ideas and facts. The staff at Hunter House have pooled their talents and skills to help me produce something that I could not have accomplished alone. They have been delightful to work with, from the first edition to this extensive third revision.

Special thanks to editor Mali Apple, for her attention to details, and for maintaining consistency and clarity. To Lisa Lee, for her ability to further manicure the manuscript and for her gentle suggestions throughout. To Paul Frindt, for turning my words into yet another good-looking book. To Corrie Sahli and Darcy Cohan, for their continued good work.

And a final thank you to my publisher and dear friend, Kiran Rana, who believed in my message long before it was in vogue.

Honorable mentions to my family, Roland, Jill, and Joey; my brother Ken; my friends, Karen, Marilyn, Darlene, and Linda, who painstakingly listened to me and supported my efforts through the sometimes grueling writing process. And to my wonderful counselor, Carole Peccorini, who introduced me to my true self and allowed me to move forward with my life's mission.

Foreword

A virtual revolution has taken place in the field of applied clinical biochemistry over the past decade. This has come about as a result of our increased recognition of the important part that nutrition plays in health. The book you now hold in your hands, *Menopause Without Medicine*, is both a testament to and an agent of this revolution.

In the past, we considered genetic inheritance the major factor in human health. In recent years, however, we have learned much more about how various nutrients modulate human biology. While our genes dictate predispositions to specific problems, the nutritional environment and our lifestyle habits alter the genetic risk. In fact, these factors may be *more* important in determining the health patterns of midlife and later age than our genes.

As a result, I believe that understanding the basics of proper nutrition and the important role it plays in the aging process is vital for everyone.

Menopause Without Medicine is a well-researched, comprehensive health guide for women approaching or going through menopause. It offers them a program to ease the transition, as well as specific nutritional remedies for common menopausal symptoms. Dr. Ojeda addresses the crucial physical problems associated with menopause: hot flashes, vaginal dryness, and osteoporosis. She explains them in terms that are easy to understand and provides sound nutritional advice for counteracting or minimizing these conditions.

Our society, focused on youth, must grow to understand that old age is not a disease. The problems we associate with aging and menopause are *not* inevitable. Dr. Ojeda lays proper stress on the necessity of preparing the body in the early years so that later symptoms will be minimal. Because she has carefully evaluated many scientific and clinical studies, and collected in one place the best of what we currently know about nutritional relief for the symptoms of menopause, the *information* in *Menopause Without Medicine* is valuable to all women.

Equally important is the author's *attitude*, which is that women must take care of their health on all fronts: physical, mental, and emotional. Her book goes beyond the physical aspects to discuss the effects of cultural attitudes and the emotions associated with menopause. In writing about issues like self-image and beauty care, sexuality and depression, Dr. Ojeda addresses the real concerns of women who want to deal positively with all the changes that accompany the climacteric.

Perhaps most important is Dr. Ojeda's *purpose* in writing this book: to empower women entering a new phase, to offer them hope and a greater measure of control over their lives. I believe *Menopause Without Medicine* is a book that can help most women in their quest for good health. It will certainly help *all* women to prepare for menopause with understanding, confidence, serenity and even, it is to be hoped, joyful anticipation.

Jeffrey S. Bland, Ph.D.

Part One

MENOPAUSE: SYMPTOMS AND REMEDIES

Introduction

Almost ten years have passed since I first started poring over medical journals searching for information about menopause—a topic that, at the time, was largely ignored by the medical community. Only a handful of books could be found on the shelves and even women's magazines omitted stories of women's experiences and dilemmas. How times have changed. Walk into any bookstore today and check out the women's health section: the racks are crammed with books on all aspects of midlife, from physical to psychological, from experiential to spiritual. Menopause is out of the closet.

As I was collecting data for the first edition of this book, I eagerly shared my findings with friends and acquaintances. It didn't take long before I realized how uncomfortable people were at the mere mention of the "M" word. Responses ranged from nervous laughter and bewilderment to downright embarrassment. I learned to lower my voice when asked how I spent my day. Only in these past few years has menopause filtered into everyday conversation. Women *and* men seem quite comfortable discussing hot flashes, mood swings, and hormone therapy. At the gym, in the office, in business meetings, in restaurants, and at parties, everyone has an opinion to offer or a story to tell.

Another noteworthy difference after a decade is that I have crossed the half-century mark. Along with my fiftieth birthday came the beginning signs of perimenopause. The symptoms that were once technical terms have taken on an entirely different meaning: hot flashes, sleepless nights, irregular periods, heart flutters, weight gain, and the decision of what to do about hormones loom over me. I find I am turning to my own words seeking remedies I discovered long ago. I am also experimenting with the new foods, nutrients, and herbs that have come to my attention since the first two editions of this book. No longer is *Menopause Without Medicine* just the product of my work as a nutritionist; it now ranks second to the Bible as my daily guide.

The perplexing issue of hormone replacement is as disturbing to me as it is to you. My knee-jerk reaction, given my nutritional science education and basic philosophy, is to reject drugs: I would rather not subject my body to potentially dangerous substances unless absolutely necessary. And isn't menopause a natural transition from one stage of life to another? If "nature" doesn't make a mistake, and we aren't meant to have children into our nineties, why should we pump hormones into our bodies when they weren't meant to be there past midlife?

I'm well aware of the potential benefits of hormone replacement therapy: lowered risk for heart disease and osteoporosis. For me—a petite, small-boned woman with a preexisting heart condition—it may be something I need to seriously reconsider. On the other hand, I exercise regularly, eat low-fat foods (most of the time), and take supplements. Personally, I feel these lifestyle measures are more conducive to preventing heart disease and osteoporosis than are hormones—and they also don't carry the risk of breast cancer or have negative side effects.

Few women's health issues are as beset with confusion and controversy as the appropriate treatment for menopause. Just using the word "treatment" suggests that menopause is a disease requiring medical care, doctor's visits, and prescription drugs. The medicalization of menopause has given birth to a giant industry composed of products, drugs, books, and nutritional supplements. Big business has discovered a dynamic market in aging baby boomers. But before you are convinced by those well-designed advertisements of vibrant, healthy midlife women popping hormones, consider the possibility that the drug companies selling these multicolored tablets for menopausal relief may not have your best interests at heart. Before you decide, read all you can about hormone replacement therapy and ask your doctor whether she or he feels it may be right for you.

Women should never blindly accept medication from a doctor without knowing what it is, what it does, and why they are taking it. And doctors should not prescribe hormones when there are no clear reasons to do so. Physicians sometimes start women on hormones prior to the onset of symptoms so they won't even know they are going through the change. Does this mean we should all take aspirin to avert a headache, or Prozac just in case depression awaits us in the future? Some women sail through menopause *without* symptoms, *without* replacement hormones, and *without* experiencing anything that requires medical care and cost.

I am not antidoctor, antimedicine, or antihormones. A hierarchy of questions and treatments needs to be considered prior to taking any drug. First, how bad is the symptom? Feeling distress at menopause does not always indicate something has gone awry. It could be a normal sign of transitioning hormones. Remember when you started your periods? For a few months you felt physically and emotionally out of sync, but your body adjusted and you eventually adapted to your new cycle. As you leave your periods in the past, there may be discomfort. If it is minimal, and if you are relieved to know it is normal, can you tolerate it without medication?

Second, are there natural, dietary, or lifestyle changes you can make to ease the symptoms? This book provides many alternatives that have been scientifically proven to work effectively for a wide variety of complaints. Nutritional and lifestyle alterations take time to pay off, but stick with them for a few months and you will see noticeable differences.

There are women for whom diet, exercise, stress reduction, and supplements aren't appropriate or do not work quickly enough. If your symptoms are intolerable and interfere with your work, relationships, and enjoyment of life, by all means get help. But even at this point, you have options. You can ask for low-potency pills, take them only as long as necessary, then slowly taper off—always in consultation with your health care provider. Many women are never informed that hormone replacement therapy doesn't have to last forever.

There is a growing appreciation of the role of nutrition in determining one's level of health. Even staunchly traditional physicians now admit that diet and lifestyle contribute to many of the major diseases. This was hardly the case 10 years ago—but there are always time lags between theory, accumulated evidence, and public awareness. It took 50 years for the medical community to indisputably link cigarette smoking to lung cancer. Decades passed before the medical establishment accepted that increased cholesterol levels were linked to heart disease. Studies showing the benefits of vitamin E in the prevention of heart disease and the treatment of hot flashes go back to the 1940s. And still I hear physicians say they need more studies before they can endorse diet and nutritional supplements as a part of health care. Given the scientific evidence and the absence of risk, waiting to inform the public that nutrients may save their lives seems irresponsible.

Nutritional and herbal remedies, as effective as they are and as much as they have been studied, do not reach the consumer to the extent that hormones and other drugs do. We are still led to believe they rank slightly higher than snake oil and placebos. Doctors on talk shows often shake their heads condescendingly when someone else brings up the validity of vitamins and herbs. We are warned more about the potential toxic effects of these concentrated food sources than we are about the potential risks of prescription drugs.

More and more we are seeing individuals taking responsibility for their own health care. According to a 1993 study, one in three Americans uses alternative therapies and pays for them out-of-pocket. The cost of health (sick) care has skyrocketed, and people are seeking less expensive methods of treatment. The concept of prevention is finally reaching public awareness: we are increasingly aware that disease may be averted with a little effort on our part.

Menopause is an exciting time—a time when we have gained a better sense of ourselves, an appreciation for the cycles of our lives, and a clearer perspective on the future. Although menopause is a universal experience, each woman goes through it in her own way and in her own time. There are many difficult decisions to make about your health, and I don't claim to have all the answers, but I do offer you some new ideas, suggestions, and thoughts on easing your immediate symptoms and improving your future years.

In making health choices, one thing I have learned is to trust my instincts. They seem to be heightened at midlife, and may offer you the truth you are seeking. Many women say, "I just *know* hormones are not for me." And they probably are not. Other women take the opposite view—with as much emotion and conviction.

I want to encourage you to feel good about whatever decision you make. Maybe you decided in advance not to take anything, but when the hot flashes kept you up for months, you reluctantly succumbed. Resist blaming yourself and others for their choices. Let us encourage each other, share our stories, learn, grow, and be happy that we live in a time when we are free to talk about women's health concerns and pass this legacy on to our daughters.

A few words about the way the book is organized: The first part deals with immediate concerns: the relief of menopausal symptoms. If you are desperately seeking a natural solution to a distressing condition, you may want to start at that specific chapter and begin your program there. The second part deals more generally with preparing for your future health, and examines risk factors for the common killers of postmenopausal women, heart disease and cancer. Becoming aware of the dietary and lifestyle factors that influence these diseases and taking action are the best insurance you have for future healthy years. I have provided outlines, questions, and charts to help you plan a course of action.

The years that follow, I believe, will be the most fulfilling, rewarding, inspiring, and fun. I know this, because every day I am more awake and alive to the reality of what life has to offer. It is my prayer that you too will see the second half as the part of life for which we have been preparing. Rehearsals are over; let the show begin.

1

MENOPAUSE: MYTH VERSUS REALITY

The woman who wants her second chance
years to be the best of all has to work
at shaping her future.
—DR. JOYCE BROTHERS,
BETTER THAN EVER

Our society today, the society in which most of us have grown up, is clearly youth-oriented. As much as we would like to believe that vitality and beauty are possible at any age, magazine ads and television commercials glaringly remind us that the emphasis on young bodies still prevails. Given our aging population and the host of beautiful older role models who now grace the screen, political arena, and corporate sector, I had begun to believe that trends might be shifting from the overwhelming focus on nubile, wrinkle-free bodies. At last maybe there will be room for more mature women. I consulted a media expert, Jan Wahl, a movie reviewer and talk show host. Jan sadly squashed my hopes: the waiflike *Vogue* model remains the American standard of female perfection.

Midlife women cannot embrace such unrealistic role models. But what is our alternative? History confronts us with an equally unsatisfying image: the pleasingly plump, matronly woman given to hysterical outbursts. She has lost her interest in looking good (forget thoughts about improving her body and mind), and no one would suggest that she is remotely interested in sex, adventure, or new experience. Neither extreme serves the 1990s menopausal woman well. Where are our role models? It appears we must be trailblazers. We must be our own role models. We must create the new image by the way we look, dress, carry ourselves, and speak the truth of this adventure. It is up to us—those of us riding the cusp of midlife—to voice our outrage at media stereotypes and to set the new standard for the modern menopausal woman.

Medical attitudes toward menopause mirror these negative stereotypes. Many earlier medical texts list it as a disease or an unnatural phenomenon. The terms most commonly used to describe it are *climacteric, endocrine starvation, involutionary years, female trouble,* and *living decay.* No wonder women tend to dread the so-called change of life. Such descriptions can significantly affect a woman's attitudes and responses to menopause, especially if she is poorly informed. Many physical and psychological reactions to menopause may be directly related to this long-term negative conditioning.

Robert Wilson, in his supposedly pro-female book *Feminine Forever,* titles one of his chapters "The Loss of Womanhood and the Loss of Good Health."[1] He describes the menopausal woman as the equivalent of a eunuch: unbearable, suicidal, incapacitated, and incapable of rationally perceiving her situation. Equally degrading is the work of David Reuben, author of the popular *Everything You Always Wanted to Know About Sex.* This "authority" maintains that the essence of femininity is tied to a woman's ovaries; once the estrogen is virtually shut off, a woman comes as close as she can to being a man. Such a woman is not really a man, he explains, but she is no longer a functional woman; according to Reuben, menopausal women live in the "world of intersex."[2] This is absurd. A woman's femininity is not defined by the amount of estrogen in her body any more than a man's masculinity is measured by his testosterone output.

The popular view of menopause is that it is a major cultural, psychological, and physiological milestone for women. The implication, however, is that it is predominately a negative event, like divorce or loss of a job. Many experts agree that menopause is a biological marker for aging: it signifies the end of reproduction in a culture where sexuality and childbearing are equated with female fulfillment, and it signifies the beginning of old age in a culture that extols youthfulness. But is this view true for all women, some women, or just a handful of menopausal women? Or is it an obsolete model reflective of antiquated ideas?

A study of over 2,500 women between the ages of 45 and 55 asked women about their real attitudes toward menopause. The most consistent message from this long-term study is that the biological event—termination of menstruation—has almost no impact on subsequent perceived physical or mental health. Furthermore, the overwhelming majority of women reported positive or neutral feelings concerning menopause.[3] It appears that the truth is that more women are either looking forward to the change or are not very concerned about it.

Also encouraging is the finding that the attitudes of women who were premenopausal at the beginning of the study and postmenopausal at completion were overwhelmingly more positive after menopause. The experience of menopause itself led to more positive and realistic attitudes.

The thought of menopause should not and need not produce anxiety. A study of other societies indicates that the stereotype of the distraught woman is not universal, that our negative reactions to common physiological processes, such as menstruation and menopause, are culturally engendered. In countries where age is venerated and elders enjoy respect for their experience and wisdom, older women seem to manifest fewer physical and psychological symptoms. For example, South African, Asian, and Arabic women, who, it is said, welcome the end of the childbearing years, are reported to have positive attitudes about the change of life. Where there are different predefined concepts, aging seems to be more natural, less confused, and not overlaid with negative images.[4]

Mayan women in Mexico have been studied by researchers because they do not complain of the characteristic symptoms of menopause and do not suffer from osteoporosis and bone fractures. Endocrinologically, they are no different from women in the United States. In fact, estrogen levels in Mayan postmenopausal women were at or below the values expected for U.S. women. Something that *is* significantly different is their attitude. Mayan women welcome the transition, as they will be relieved of many household chores and regarded as respected elders. In addition, they will be free from the taboos associated with menstruation. Menstruating women are believed to carry an "evil wind" during their periods, so cessation of periods raises a woman's status in the community.[5]

Menopause, like menarche, is natural. We will experience hormonal changes at menopause just as we did in our adolescence. Any lifetime change may be accompanied by uneasiness and disequilibrium; it is normal and it will pass. How smoothly a woman adapts to any transition depends largely on her overall health: her body, her mind, and her spirit.

MENOPAUSE IS BIG BUSINESS

Historically, the menopausal woman was regarded with pity and indifference. Because she complained of symptoms that were as yet unexplained, she was labeled a neurotic hypochondriac, then sedated and left to suffer in silence. I am sure no one regrets leaving behind those days of disbelief and intolerance. But what replaced the ignorance—the new medical model of midlife—may be equally destructive.

Women who are 50-something are no longer ignored; they are actively courted. They are presently a prime target of the medical institution, drug companies, and other interests that can benefit from an aging population. And the market is growing: the number of women aged 45 to 54 is expected to jump 50 percent between 1990 and 2000. Over the next decade about 1.2 million women annually will become menopausal. Talk about global warming.

Industry-financed medical researchers inundate us with information about the benefits of treating all menopausal signs and symptoms, severe or insignificant, with hormones. While earlier hormonal therapies were marketed only to physicians, major drug companies now directly target female consumers in the grocery store magazines. Before they experience their first hint of oncoming menopause, women are primed to run to the doctor for pills.

Menopause is now a big business and we women consumers need to be alert to what we hear and read. The fact that there is a strong bias toward medicalizing menopause is obvious. Hormone replacement therapy (HRT) may be beneficial and the proper choice for some women; the tendency, however, is to offer women HRT as their only option and not notify them about the potential dangers and side effects. Before *you* make a decision about your plan of action, get a balanced perspective by reading as much as you can from medical and nonmedical sources. Women who are taking pills for no known reason may benefit from reading *The Menopause Industry* by Sandra Coney. *The Estrogen Decision* by Susan Lark considers both sides of the question. Another way of informing yourself about the latest in health reform is to join the National Women's Health Network. Their monthly newsletter reviews the most current information to date. Other books and newsletters are listed in the Resources section of this book.

Women must understand the workings of their bodies, with all of the hormonal fluctuations, to avoid unnecessary fear, anxiety, and stress. Understanding can also enhance a woman's experience of her changing body. It is time to shed the myths and misconceptions about menopause that our society has harbored and to build a foundation for the sense of well-being that each woman deserves.

THE RANGE OF SYMPTOMS

I was raised in an era when normal female topics, such as menstruation and menopause, were not openly discussed even among close friends. Our bodies, we were led to believe, were too mysterious to understand and too base to mention. Our intimate parts were ignored as if they did not exist. Even today, unfortunately, these childhood attitudes linger, preventing many of us from confronting and accepting problems and feelings that cry out to be addressed.

Attitudes concerning the menopause experience have changed in the last few years, and they continue to evolve as women read, learn, and discuss their individual experiences. Recently, a questionnaire designed by Fredi Kronenberg, director of menopause research at the Center for Women's Health at Columbia-Presbyterian Medical Center, New York City, was given to readers of *Prevention* magazine.[6] The results of the 2,000 randomly chosen respondents (15,000 actually provided information) may help us understand

and appreciate the menopausal experience. The results of this extensive questionnaire include the following:

+ Intensity of symptoms ranged from stormy to breezy. Fifty-eight percent considered the process more of an annoyance than a major life disruption, and more than half agreed the symptoms were, for the most part, mild.

+ The younger the age of menopause, the more difficult the experience. The average age at the onset of menopause is 50 years, and a woman who has, for example, postponed motherhood thinking she still has 10 years left, and then suddenly finds herself starting menopause probably has both physical and psychological issues to confront.

+ Weight gain is not inevitable at 50; however, 42 percent of respondents gained in excess of 10 pounds. Current research indicates that this additional poundage is more a function of aging than of estrogen decline.

+ The fact that sleep problems were prevalent was not surprising. Sixty-two percent of the respondents reported that hot flashes kept them awake. Frequent urination, which is related to lower estrogen levels, may also keep women awake; aging itself has an effect on muscle tone, and illnesses such as diabetes impact bladder function.

+ The years prior to menopause, perimenopause, seem to account for most of the annoying symptoms, such as severe hormonal fluctuations. Once a woman has stopped having periods for a year, things usually stabilize.

+ Good health habits correlated with a more positive menopausal experience. Exercising three or more times a week was associated with fewer symptoms and a generally better transition. It is unclear whether exercise reduced the stress of menopause or had other benefits, but the more stress a woman reported in her life, the more difficult her menopause.

+ The relationship between a positive menopause experience and a low-fat diet was even stronger than that for exercise.

Women who described their diet as primarily vegetarian generally reported fewer symptoms. Eating soy products such as tofu correlated strongly with fewer symptoms. It may be that women who eat soy and vegetable products have a lifestyle that is healthier in other ways, but the benefit might also be attributed to the large amounts of *phytohormones* in soy. Certain plants have estrogenlike properties that appear to provide just enough hormone to prevent menopausal symptoms. In countries where women consume large amounts of soy products, menopausal symptoms are appreciably reduced or nonexistent.

PERSONALITY TYPES

It appears that women with certain personalities may tend to develop certain menopausal symptoms. Although the evidence is not conclusive, there is value in relaying this information, because it may apply to and help a number of women.

Researchers have found that certain personality types find it more traumatic to adjust to changes during the menopausal years. Gynecologist Sheldon Cherry finds that women with a history of emotional problems have the hardest time. These include women with chronic sexual difficulties, immature women with narcissistic tendencies, women whose erotic attractiveness was the chief element of their personal worth, childless women facing the undeniable loss of fertility, and married women who feel that their meaningful years are over.[7]

Several authorities have observed that the manner in which women react to the change may be related to how they perceive themselves as women. Particularly vulnerable, according to British physician Barbara Evans, are women who over the years have defined their femininity in terms of bodily functions—menstruation, pregnancy—and motherhood.[8] For them, menopause represents the end of their womanly identity; it removes the purpose of their existence.

Another all-too-common phenomenon is women who submerge their own desires, talents, and personal growth to live totally through their children's activities and accomplishments. It is no wonder that, when their children leave home, these women undergo an emotional trauma similar to experiencing the death of a loved one. They have lost the chief component of their identity as women and as a contributing member of society. This "empty-nest syndrome" often results in depression. The midlife woman must search for a new identity in her relationship to her grown children.

The degree to which a woman accepts or fears growing older also affects the transition. The reality of getting older has to be dealt with at some time in our lives, and often this time coincides with or begins at menopause. If the thought of aging, coupled with diminishing attractiveness and usefulness, frightens you, I would like to recommend a book I find particularly inspiring. In *Always a Woman*, Kaylan Pickford, a successful New York fashion model who happens to be over 50, emphasizes the beauty to be found in all phases of life. No one part is better or to be compared to another, she tells us; each is unique and special. "While there can be beauty in life that is in the process of becoming (as in a flower bud), there is also beauty in life that has achieved itself (as in the flower in full bloom)."[9]

Research indicates that women who accept menopause as a natural passage in life are likely to get through it unscathed. For them, the transition is comparatively uncomplicated, uneventful, and relatively symptomless. In addition, women whose educational skills make more options available to them are reported to handle the change with relative ease.[10] Numerous studies indicate that women with professional interests, intellectual and creative outlets, and challenging responsibilities have an easier time during menopause. It is not clear exactly why active women appear to suffer less physical and emotional pain than their homebound sisters, but theories are that they have less time to focus on their symptoms, are generally more knowledgeable about the physiological details of menopause and about their own bodies, and have higher self-esteem.

Whether a woman's symptoms during menopause will be closely related to her personality type or feelings about herself cannot be predicted with any certainty. To portray such a complex psychophysiological process in black-and-white terms would be misleading. Each woman has a highly individual chemical makeup,

genetic predisposition, and hormonal balance. Even the most secure, well-adjusted, and happy woman may experience emotional
upheaval during menopause. Fortunately, the majority of women
not only accept the multiple challenges of menopause, but find it
to be the most enriching time of their lives.

CREATING A POSITIVE IMAGE

Women entering menopause are approaching what can be the best
years of their lives. The life span of the modern woman is currently
78 years, and gerontologists anticipate that it will soon increase to 80.
Even the conservative American Medical Association's Council on
Medical Services boldly asserts that with intelligent living we
could all live to be 90 or 100 years old. This means that, before
too many more decades have passed, the average woman may be
living as many years after menopause as she lived before it. We
need to be concerned with enhancing the quality of those years.
Just think: if a woman has devoted the first half or third of her life
to raising a family, she can still return to college, start a new
career, travel, write the great American novel, learn French, or
climb Mount Everest. We don't have to restrict ourselves to one
career or one life path. Our options increase, especially when we
are mentally and physically prepared to exercise them.

In spite of the opportunities menopause opens up for us, we
should not underestimate the emotional impact menopause has on
many women. Psychologist Helene Deutsch calls the psychological
experience of menopause the most trying time of a woman's life,
and Juanita Williams agrees: "Although it is the manifest sign of
the end of reproductive life, its symbolic meanings invest it with
an importance which extends far beyond its biological definition."[11]
Whether this applies to you is not something a textbook or expert
can predict—only you can say. If menopause represents more than
a physical change to you, find a support group where you are free
to discuss your feelings openly. By working through these issues
with others, you may find they become much more manageable.

Psychological research has shown that a person's behavior
can be affected by her expectations, and that expectations can become
a self-fulfilling prophecy. Examine your own cultural associations

and belief systems concerning menopause. Are they based on fact or fallacy? Listed below are my responses to the most common misconceptions about menopause. What are your feelings about them?

+ Menopause is not the beginning of the end.

+ You will not age faster after menopause.

+ You do not have to gain weight, become depressed, or lose your looks because of lowered estrogen levels.

+ Fertility does not equal femininity.

+ You do not lose interest in sex because of decreasing estrogen.

+ Taking estrogen will not keep you young.

+ Your feelings are just as genuine at menopause as at any other time of your life.

+ Menopause is not mysterious; the process is easy to understand.

+ Medication is not the answer to all menopausal symptoms.

+ You do not have to suffer in silence; in fact, you do not have to suffer at all.

What we think and believe not only determines our daily decisions, it also establishes the entire direction of our life. Attitudes shape our future. If you have accepted an idea—from yourself, a teacher, parent, friend, an advertisement, or any other source —and, if you are firmly convinced that idea is true, it has the same power over you as a hypnotist's words have over the hypnotist's subject.[12] We translate into physical reality the thoughts and attitudes we hold in our minds, no matter what they are.

Our attitudes toward menopause may have been engendered by our culture and our families, but they are not unchangeable. If our ideas are counterproductive, we can choose to acknowledge the fears and anxieties we harbor and alter them, and begin to reverse the obstacles in our lives.

Whether you are 50 years old or 20, take stock of your belief system and your general attitudes. If you feel you are valued only for your children's or husband's accomplishments, then few can know and acknowledge the real you. If you think that to be beautiful you must be young, your mature years will have little joy. If you are convinced that the quality of your life will vanish at 50 or 60 or 70, it will. If you believe your health, looks, body, and mind all begin to deteriorate with the onset of menopause, they probably will.

We women are often experts at suppressing our innermost thoughts. We have learned through years of conditioning to keep up appearances and to insist that everything is fine when our bodies and souls silently scream the opposite. We try so hard to please our children, parents, friends, and neighbors, to be all they would like us to be, that we lose sight of who we are and what we believe. We try to become everything to everyone, yet end up being nothing to ourselves. We carry around vestiges of ancient traditions, obsolete fears, and borrowed beliefs, promising that some day when life is less hectic we will sort everything out; and we lose touch with our inner selves.

Menopause is a time in life when many women rediscover themselves, the self that somehow lost its way in the midst of raising a family, earning a living, and doing life. The process may not be easy, but the rewards of rediscovering yourself can make the journey tremendously worthwhile. Be kind to yourself as you travel this road, and allow your instinct to direct your course.

In the following chapters, I will discuss aspects of menopause and aging, as well as understanding and taking charge of our bodies. The first step in taking charge of our bodies is taking charge of our lives. I will tell you how to prepare, how to cope, how to eliminate many problems, and how to make the most of what nature has given you. The rest should be much easier.

2

THE PHYSICAL REALITY

We have lived through the era when
happiness was a warm puppy, and the
era when happiness was a dry martini,
and now we have come to the era when
happiness is "knowing what your
uterus looks like."

—NORA EPHRON

The word *menopause* is derived from two Greek roots: *mens*, meaning monthly, and *pause*, meaning to stop. It refers to the cessation of menstruation and the termination of fertility, events that don't necessarily happen at the same time. The time of a woman's final menstrual period can only be determined retrospectively. When a woman has not had periods for one year, she is said to have passed through menopause and is officially *postmenopausal*.

The span of time before the last period is *perimenopause*. It may extend anywhere from a few months to several years and is characterized by irregular periods and other symptoms such as hot flashes, changes in sleeping patterns, fatigue, heart palpitations, vaginal dryness, mood swings, and weight gain. The number, degree, and intensity of symptoms vary from woman to woman.

Terminology describing the ovarian and hormonal transitions associated with menopause has changed in the past several years. At one time *climacteric*, considered the counterpart of puberty, referred to the entire menopause process from the first sign to the last period. It is seldom seen in print anymore, and I personally don't miss it. The word connotes climax and finality. While it is true that menstruation ceases, menopause is far from being the climax of a woman's life.

The *change of life* or *the change* find their way into the literature to encompass the diversity of the entire midlife experience: physical, emotional, and spiritual. They are vague terms, and appropriately so: each woman defines them as she sees them applying to her.

WHEN WILL IT BEGIN?

For most American women today, the termination of fertility usually takes place between 48 and 52 years of age. Interestingly, the mean age of menopause has increased by approximately four years over the past century, and gynecologists report that many women are still menstruating well into their sixth decade.[1] Improved nutrition, healthier lifestyles, and modern medical advances are the most notable reasons for this increase in childbearing years. This news may be encouraging to women who have postponed having children. Many factors influence whether menopause will arrive early or late, and these are discussed below.

✦ **Lifestyle**   Several studies have examined the effect of lifestyle on the onset of menopause. Nutrition in particular appears to be a significant factor. An extensive survey conducted in New Guinea found that undernourished women start menopause around the age of 43, while those more adequately nourished do not begin until age 47.[2] Research on large population groups indicates that European women, who supposedly engage in healthier habits than Americans, tend toward a later menopause.

✦ **Nature and nurture**   Heredity must always be taken into account. There is some indication that women tend to follow in their mothers' footsteps: if the mother had a late menopause, the daughter's may be late as well. But is this nature or nurture? A growing number of scientists believe that the influence is cultural rather than genetic. Children tend to imitate their parents' habits: how much they exercise, how and what they eat, how they handle stress, and whether they smoke cigarettes or drink alcohol. These environmental factors may be at least as important as inherited tendencies.

✦ **Smoking**   The data from two large, independent studies involving several countries have confirmed that smokers generally experience earlier menopause. There are two probable explanations for this finding: first, nicotine, which acts on the central nervous system, may decrease the secretion of hormones; second, nicotine may activate liver-metabolizing enzymes that alter the metabolization of the sex-related hormones.[3]

✦ **Trauma**   A traumatic experience may trigger early or premature menopause. Premature menopause occurs when periods stop permanently before the age of 40. Early menopause may start any time before the normal age range of 48 to 52. Prolonged stress or a crisis can temporarily halt the production of certain hormones, and the ovaries, responding to the lack of these hormones, may cease production of eggs, and subsequently of estrogen and progesterone. Periods stop and typical menopausal symptoms appear. This *traumatic menopause* should not be confused with *psychogenic amenorrhea*, which is a temporary cessation of periods caused by tension, fatigue, exercise, low body weight, or malnutrition. If an underweight woman stops menstruating because of an inadequate amount of body fat, she will usually resume her normal cycle shortly after her weight returns to normal. In other words, psychogenic amenorrhea is most often temporary; this is not generally the case for women going through premature or traumatic menopause.

✦ **Continuous low body weight**   Women who have been undernourished for long periods of time are likely to go through menopause several years earlier than the norm. If a woman's body weight remains unnaturally low to the point of anorexia, it is possible that the ovaries will shut down permanently, resulting in premature menopause. Women in their 30s and even some in their 20s have ended their child-bearing years through self-starvation.

✦ **Oophorectomy and hysterectomy**   When a woman's ovaries are irreparably damaged or when she has them surgically removed (*ovariectomy* or *oophorectomy*), she will begin menopause immediately. This operation should not be confused with a *hysterectomy*, the removal of the uterus alone. Many women are under the impression that after a hysterectomy, the change is imminent. However, though the woman will no longer have periods or be capable of becoming pregnant, if one or both ovaries—or even only part of one—is left intact, eggs and female hormones will continue to be produced until menopause occurs.[4] A hysterectomy can, however, result in an early menopause, perhaps even by several years.[5] Early menopause is a possibility whenever the blood circulation is cut off or compromised in any way, such as during sterilization by tubal ligation or from damage caused by radiation treatment, chemotherapy, and certain diseases.

I would like to digress for a moment. There is considerable controversy today about unnecessary hysterectomy or ovariectomy. Because women have frequently accepted medical recommendations without asking questions or seeking second opinions, they have often been victims of unnecessary surgery. Studies estimate that from 15 percent to 60 percent of all such operations are unnecessary. It has been projected that within the next several years, gynecological surgeons will have removed over one half of the uteruses in the United States. Will all these operations be performed for valid reasons? Many concerned health advocates think not.

The decision to have one's female organs removed is a serious one. Several books offer guidelines on when hysterectomies may be indicated, and when they are normally performed but are not compulsory. If you are faced with this question, begin by gathering as much information as you can, pro and con. For an excellent discussion of this subject, I recommend *The New Our Bodies, Ourselves*, by the Boston Women's Health Book Collective. Ask your physician why surgery is indicated, what exactly is to be removed, what your alternatives are, and what the future implications are. Do not be afraid to ask these questions—it is *your*

Factors That May Influence the Timing of the Onset of Menopause

EARLIER	LATER
. . . . . . genetics	
. . . . . . stress	
. . . . . . drugs.	
underweight	overweight
hysterectomy	cancer of breast or uterus
tubal ligation	fibroids
damaged female organs	diabetes
smoking	
malnutrition	

body. Once you are clear about the basis for the diagnosis, get a second opinion. Before you go ahead, make sure you are satisfied this is the right choice for you. If surgery is unavoidable (and it may be your *only* option), prepare emotionally and nutritionally to minimize any aftereffects. A healthy mind and a strong body are the best guarantees for a smooth operation and a quick recovery.

Now, let's return to the factors that affect the onset of menopause. As discussed, when estrogen is diminished in any way, menopause is likely to begin early. The biological clock may also operate in reverse: should the premenopausal supply of estrogen continue as usual, the process will be delayed.

✦ Excess body fat   One common condition that can *delay* menopause is an excess of body fat. Overweight women menstruate longer than their thinner sisters because their bodies manufacture greater amounts of estrogen. Estrogen is produced not only in the ovaries, but also in the fatty tissues of the body from another hormone, androstenedione. The more fat a woman carries, the more estrogen she makes. I suppose this could be construed as one "natural" way to postpone menopause, but it is certainly not the wisest. For one thing, an overabundance of circulating estrogen increases the risk of estrogen-based cancers. Having a little extra padding is not a worry and may minimize symptoms, but, as in all things, more is not necessarily better.

Other Physical Problems

Certain diseases have been known to provoke the endocrine system into extending estrogen production. Although the evidence is not conclusive, physicians have observed that women with cancer of the breast and uterus, women with fibroids, and women who are diabetic may expect menopause to come somewhat later than average.

WHO EXPERIENCES SYMPTOMS?

It has been estimated that 75 to 80 percent of women passing through menopause experience one or more symptoms, but only 10 to 35 percent are affected strongly enough to seek professional help. While it is impossible to predict who will suffer severe symptoms, certain generalizations can be made.[6]

Characteristics of Women Likely to Pass Through Menopause Undisturbed

✦ relatively late onset of menstruation

✦ never been married

✦ never been pregnant

✦ gave birth after age 40

✦ relatively high income

✦ better educated

Characteristics of Women Likely to Suffer Severe Menopausal Symptoms

✦ premenstrual syndrome sufferer

✦ had premature menopause

✦ had artificial menopause (oophorectomy)

It is obvious from the above lists that physiology is only one piece of the menopausal puzzle—and probably the easiest part to understand. Why should women who have never been married or who have had a child after 40 be less likely to experience these symptoms? Is there another underlying common denominator—lifestyle, education, diet—that might explain these parallels? Future research must address these questions.

Generally, the *rate* at which estrogen levels drop influences the number and severity of symptoms. Usually, these follow one of three patterns:

✦ **Pattern A: Abrupt ending**   This is the immediate cessation of menstrual periods, where periods stop without prior warning. It is fairly uncommon; in most cases, the ovaries stop functioning gradually. If the estrogen supply stops suddenly, the chances of experiencing symptoms are greater. However, not all women follow the norm. Menopause researcher Rosetta Reitz found a group whose periods stopped abruptly, yet who complained of relatively few symptoms.[7] She presumed these women had a high threshold for discomfort. This suggests that, while there are definable patterns, it is difficult to predict how any one woman will go through the change.

✦ **Pattern B: Gradual ending**   This is a more common occurrence, involving a progressive decline in both the amount and duration of the menstrual flow. Typically, periods become shorter, delayed, or skipped; finally, they terminate altogether. A woman may not even be aware of the irregularity of her cycles. If the ovaries atrophy slowly, if the organs they stimulate are not hypersensitive, and if they continue to supply a sustaining amount of estrogen, symptoms are insignificant.[8]

✦ **Pattern C: Irregular ending**   Irregular menstrual patterns are also relatively common. The flow may be sporadic; it may become heavier, lighter, or alternate monthly. The number of days between periods may increase or decrease. Some women may go an entire year without one period, and then, without warning, start menstruating again. Many "change-of-life babies" have been born because women thought they were safe. Doctors now urge women to continue birth control for two years after their last period.

Numerous researchers, searching for possible relationships among roles, behavior, and a tendency toward menopausal distress, have found that a psychological component is clearly involved in menopausal distress.[9] How much of a woman's discomfort is physical and how much is a response to cultural expectations and her own belief system is difficult to determine. Each woman's symptoms and physical reactions may be genuine and yet nothing like those of her friends.

THE MENSTRUAL CYCLE

To have a good understanding of the ways in which a woman's body changes from age 40 to age 60, it helps to have a clear understanding of the menstrual cycle. Even in this age of health consciousness and fitness, too many women do not know what is occurring monthly in their bodies. Understanding how your body

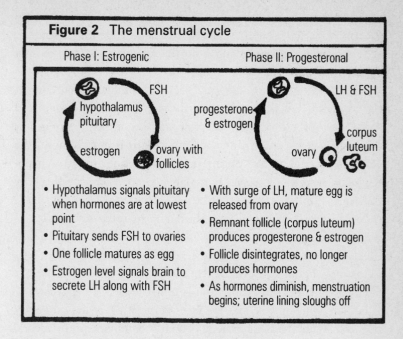

Figure 2 The menstrual cycle

Phase I: Estrogenic

Phase II: Progesteronal

- Hypothalamus signals pituitary when hormones are at lowest point
- Pituitary sends FSH to ovaries
- One follicle matures as egg
- Estrogen level signals brain to secrete LH along with FSH

- With surge of LH, mature egg is released from ovary
- Remnant follicle (corpus luteum) produces progesterone & estrogen
- Follicle disintegrates, no longer produces hormones
- As hormones diminish, menstruation begins; uterine lining sloughs off

works is critical to taking charge of your health and your life. Even if you believe you understand the process of menstruation, please read this section carefully—you may increase your body awareness.

The female menstrual cycle is the 28- or 29-day period that repeats itself monthly for a woman's fertile life. It involves an interplay among the brain, the ovaries, and four primary hormones, two secreted at each location (see Figure 2). The release of these hormones primarily stimulates the cells lining the uterus in preparation for a possible pregnancy. The uterine lining, or *endometrium*, is built up in the first part of the cycle and shed during the menstrual period.

A cycle has no beginning or end, but for the purpose of explanation we will start with the physical stages of the menstrual cycle at the *hypothalamus*, an endocrine gland in the brain. Commonly referred to as the master controller, the hypothalamus plays a key role in many basic bodily functions such as regulating body temperature, water balance, metabolic rate, appetite, sleep patterns, and tolerance to stress. The hypothalamus sends a message in the form of a hormone to the *anterior pituitary gland*, another endocrine gland located just below it. The tiny pituitary responds to the message by secreting the first hormone of the cycle, called *follicle-stimulating hormone* (FSH). Like all endocrine hormones, FSH is a messenger traveling from one organ to act on another part of the body; in this case, the ovaries.

Within the ovaries are small sacs called follicles that contain eggs and the female hormone, estrogen. Stimulation from FSH causes one of the follicles to grow and, as it does, estrogen is released. When a specific amount of estrogen is circulating in the bloodstream, the pituitary, again under instructions from the hypothalamus, secretes its second hormone, *luteinizing hormone* (LH). By this time, the egg is mature and ready to burst from the follicle.

The egg is expelled into the fallopian tubes and makes its way up into the uterus. The actual release of the egg is called *ovulation*, and it marks roughly the halfway point in the cycle. Remaining behind in the ovary, the remnant follicle is now a functioning endocrine gland, and is now called the *corpus luteum*. It is the corpus luteum that produces both estrogen and progesterone, the second female hormone, which is dominant in the second half of the cycle. The varying levels of the four hormones active in a typical menstrual cycle are shown in Figure 3.

If the egg is fertilized by a sperm, it implants or attaches to the lining of the uterus and a special hormone called *chorionic gonadotropin* is secreted. This hormone stimulates the continued secretion of estrogen and progesterone so that the developing embryo will be nourished. Without fertilization of the egg and continued hormonal production, the corpus luteum shrivels and dies, and estrogen and progesterone secretion drops. When both hormones reach their lowest point, the thickened uterine lining is sloughed off through the vaginal opening and menstrual flow begins. Low blood levels of estrogen and progesterone act as a signal to the brain to produce FSH, and the whole process starts again.

During the cycle, estrogen's primary function is to increase the blood supply and thus thicken the endometrium in preparation for a suitable environment for fertilization, implantation, and nutrition of the embryo. Progesterone further prepares the uterus for reception and development of the fertilized ovum by making available an adequate supply of nutrients.

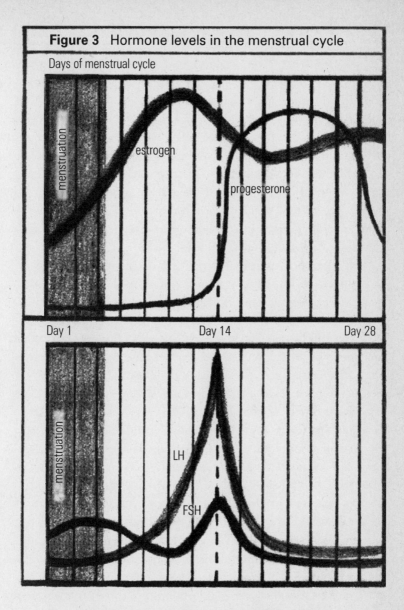

Figure 3 Hormone levels in the menstrual cycle

Days of menstrual cycle

menstruation

estrogen

progesterone

Day 1   Day 14   Day 28

menstruation

LH

FSH

CHANGES AT MENOPAUSE

The first indication of approaching menopause is the beginning of *anovulatory cycles*, that is, cycles in which ovulation does not take place. Ovarian function actually begins to decline several years prior to menopause. The follicles that inhabit the ovaries gradually diminish in number from birth, reducing the initial 250,000 potential eggs to approximately 50 by age 40 and eventually none after menopause. With fewer follicles, some months may pass when menstruation does not occur. No follicle means no egg, no estrogen, no corpus luteum, no progesterone, and no period (see Figure 4). As the ovaries continue to reduce their production of estrogen and progesterone, the pituitary gland, in a desperate effort to stimulate the recalcitrant ovaries, pumps greater amounts of FSH and LH into the blood. FSH escalates, reaching levels 13 times that of normal cycles, while LH levels rise approximately three-fold.[10] As explained to me by gynecologist Larry Francis, this elevation of hormones is most commonly and easily used by physicians to test for the onset of menopause.

In the perimenopausal period, the levels of the brain hormones increase while the ovarian hormone levels decrease. When the ovaries stop producing eggs, progesterone, which depends on a corpus luteum for production, is no longer secreted. Estrogen, however, can still be manufactured by the ovaries (although in smaller amounts), by the adrenal glands, and by extraglandular sources (including certain fat cells). During the premenopausal stage, the uterine lining is being stimulated exclusively by estrogen. With no periodic shedding of the uterine lining, the tissues continue to proliferate until the lining outgrows its blood-vessel supply. It may be several months before this happens; thus, periods are often missed or irregular. When it does break down and disintegrate, it often comes off haphazardly, in uneven patches, resulting in a heavier than normal period.

Ultimately, the ovarian follicles no longer respond to the prodding of FSH and LH. Estrogen levels drop too low to cause growth in the uterine lining, menstruation ceases completely, and menopause begins. Although the mature ovary no longer ovulates, it has not ceased functioning altogether. In fact, the central region of the ovary is actively engaged in producing hormones that are converted into *estrone*, the form of estrogen that remains circulating in the blood after menopause. Tests have shown that some women show significant evidence of estrogenic activity more than 20 years after their last period.[11] Usually, the adrenal glands become the major source of postmenopausal estrogen. In fact, main-

Figure 4 Premenopausal menstrual cycles

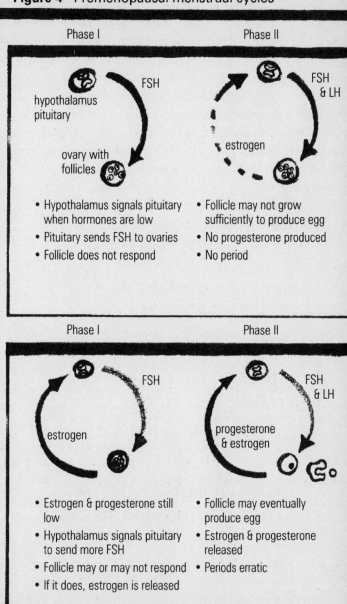

Phase I

- Hypothalamus signals pituitary when hormones are low
- Pituitary sends FSH to ovaries
- Follicle does not respond

Phase II

- Follicle may not grow sufficiently to produce egg
- No progesterone produced
- No period

Phase I

- Estrogen & progesterone still low
- Hypothalamus signals pituitary to send more FSH
- Follicle may or may not respond
- If it does, estrogen is released

Phase II

- Follicle may eventually produce egg
- Estrogen & progesterone released
- Periods erratic

taining healthy adrenals may be one of the best ways to ensure continued estrogen production and a smoother transition.

Estrone is also converted in the body fat from another hormone, *androstenedione*. As was mentioned earlier, women with ample fat on their bodies not only experience menopause later because of higher estrogen levels; they also appear to suffer less discomfort than their thinner sisters. The conversion of androstenedione into estrone has been found to occur in the muscle, liver, kidney, brain, and possibly other unknown extraglandular sources.[12] Clearly, as the ovaries slow down, the production of estrogen diminishes, but the body readjusts, substituting other estrogen sources.

What Happens to the Hormones at Menopause

✦ Ovarian activity decreases.
   Estrogen is produced in decreased amounts.
   Progesterone is no longer secreted.

✦ Brain hormones temporarily increase.
   FSH and LH are produced in greater amounts.

✦ Estrone is produced from various sources:
   adrenal glands,
   body fat,
   extraglandular sources, and
   ovaries.

PHYSIOLOGICAL CHANGES FOLLOWING MENOPAUSE

Estrogen is of primary importance in the female life cycle. The amount of estrogen circulating in the body, its ratio to other hormones, and its rate of change and decline prior to menopause all have effects on physical health and emotional outlook. Estrogen acts directly on the uterus, and influences other organs and tissues such as the vulva, vagina, breasts, bones, hair, skin, heart, and central nervous system. As the level of estrogen decreases, substantial changes occur in the appearance and function of all these organs. This is not to say that every menopausal symptom is related to declining hormones—some are the natural results of aging. For example, hot flashes, the loss of vaginal lubrication, and thinning of tissues are probably hormonally dependent, while the loss of elasticity, middle-age spread, and sagging skin are probably not.

Postmenopausal women experience varying degrees of *atrophic* (shrinking and thinning) changes of the vagina, cervix, uterus, and ovaries. Most women can expect a decrease in the size of the cervix and uterus, accompanied by a reduction in cervical mucus. Some women become more prone to bacterial infections because of the decline in cervical secretions. The *labia majora* (larger skin folds of the vagina) become thinner, flatter, paler, and less elastic. The vaginal wall shortens and loses its muscle tone as well as some of its normal secretions, sometimes making intercourse uncomfortable or painful.

Structures around the reproductive organs suffer loss of muscle tone as a result of natural aging and lack of exercise. In the extreme state, the relaxed structures fall into other organs. For example, the uterus may fall, causing the cervix to rest on or even enter the vaginal wall. A sensation of heaviness in the vaginal area or the feeling that tissue is protruding outward may indicate a descending bladder, uterus, or rectum. Lack of muscle tone may also cause the urinary sphincter muscles not to contract satisfactorily, so that urine escapes when the individual laughs, sneezes, coughs, or lifts heavy objects. Uncontrollable urinary leaking (incontinence) can be prevented or relieved through special exercises called Kegel exercises, described in Chapter 5.

Fat disappears from the breast tissue, reducing the breasts' size, shape, and firmness. Nipples tend to become smaller and less erect. Some women report decreased sexual stimulation from the breast, but whether this is physical or psychological is undetermined. On the positive side, women who have been tormented by fibrocystic breast disease (lumpy, painful breasts) will be relieved to know that this discomfort usually subsides during or after menopause.

Aging also creates obvious changes in the hair and skin. Body hair may thin out in some women and increase in others. New growth on the upper lip and chin is ascribed to the reversed ratio of estrogen to androgen. While women always have this "male" hormone in their systems, it is only after menopause that it is physically discernible.

Wrinkling and loss of skin tone are particularly noticeable around the face, neck, and hands. Characteristic purse-string wrinkles form around the mouth and "crows' feet" develop at the corners of the eyes. Natural preventive measures can minimize at least some fine aging lines.

There is a pervasive belief that women who take estrogen therapy or use estrogen creams appear younger; this is debatable. In an informal survey, Barbara Seaman and Gideon Seaman observed that estrogen users did not look more youthful; they only thought they did. On the other hand, women who did not rely on hormone therapy but were very conscientious about diet and exercise were (in the Seamans' opinion) young in appearance.[13] These well-respected researchers concluded that estrogen therapy may give women a false sense of security and prevent them from engaging in commonsense approaches to aging.

For many years, women passively accepted the "matronly" image of aging: as women get older, their body configuration alters, fat redistributes, the metabolism slows down, and there is a tendency to gain weight. That image is changing. With a little conscious effort, regular exercise, and fewer calories, women are working to maintain healthy, trim, and toned figures throughout their lives.

When hormone levels fall, the bones tend to lose density. Reduced estrogen activity has been directly related to accelerated bone loss, which explains why osteoporosis, the world's most common bone disease, is rampant in postmenopausal women. Loss of bone mass is believed by many researchers to account for the prevalence of hip and vertebral fractures as well as the hunched-over posture of some older women. All women should be particularly aware that diet and exercise—especially in the early adult years—are keys to preventing this crippling disease.

Clearly, estrogen is vital to the female body. When we produce too much or too little, symptoms occur. However, even though more than 50 symptoms have been attributed to the endocrine changes that occur during the change—tiredness, nervousness, headaches, irritability, depression, insomnia, joint and muscle pain, dizziness, heart palpitation, breathlessness, and impatience, among others—a direct cause-and-effect relationship for each has not been clearly determined. Ovarian decline and diminished estrogen levels are hardly the only factors to consider. More important may be the overall health of the individual and her ability to adapt to the transitions taking place in her organ systems and in her life.

Physical Changes at Midlife

+ Some atrophying of vagina, cervix, uterus, and ovaries takes place.

+ Vaginal wall shortens, thins out, and loses muscle tone.

+ Labia majora become thinner, paler, and less elastic.

+ Supporting structures (sphincter muscles, bladder, rectum) lose muscle tone.

+ Secretion of cervical mucus is reduced.

+ Breast size, firmness, and shape changes.

+ Body hair gets thinner in most women; in some, it increases.

+ Wrinkling and loss of skin tone occur.

+ Body fat is redistributed.

+ Bone mass is lost.

+ Metabolic rate slows.

The following chapters discuss in more detail specific symptoms and problems associated with menopause. Remember that, for the most part, suffering through severe symptoms is neither normal nor necessary. In most cases, a commonsense approach to nutrition, regular exercise, and an otherwise healthy lifestyle are the only "medication" you will need.

3

Hot Flashes

A flush is anything but a flash.
—JOHN W. STUDD, MRCOG
KING'S COLLEGE HOSPITAL, LONDON

The most characteristic complaint of menopause is the bothersome hot flash, more correctly called hot *flush*. Up to 80 percent of women experience them to some degree, with up to 40 percent suffering enough to seek medical attention. Some women never have a hot flash, most are inconvenienced for a year or two, and for a few, flashes may persist up to 5, even 10 years.

Hot flashes usually begin when periods are still regular or are just starting to fluctuate, and are often one of the first indications that menopause is approaching. Generally, they are most uncomfortable in the first stages of perimenopause, gradually decreasing in frequency and intensity as the body adapts to the hormonal changes.

Descriptions of a hot flash are as varied as the personalities of the women having them. Mine started with an immediate surge of heat enveloping my body from head to foot, as if someone had suddenly turned the thermostat way up. It happened regularly every night and in the early mornings for about three months, then gradually tapered off. The discomfort was minimal, but the interrupted sleep made me grouchy and groggy. It felt like a permanent case of jet lag. A friend described a wave of heat that began in her face and neck and worked down to her chest. She turned scarlet, perspired profusely, then shivered for several minutes. Changing her nightgown and sheets was a nightly ritual. Her experience seemed to take a great toll on her emotional health. Crying spells, panic attacks, and eating binges also disrupted her daily activities.

Flashes differ in duration, frequency, and intensity. Episodes may be brief—two to three minutes—but can also linger up to an hour. They can come several times a day or night, or only once or twice a week.

In itself, the hot flash is harmless. Nevertheless, as the body's temperature control system vacillates between very hot and cool, other body systems are strained as well. When flashes occur too often, they may be accompanied by unexpected and even frightening side effects: loss of sleep, fatigue, weakness, dizziness, a racing pulse, heart palpitations, headaches, itchy skin, and numbness in the hands and arms. These symptoms can take you unaware and cause concern as thoughts of more serious causes race through your mind.

WHAT CAUSES HOT FLASHES?

The hot flash is still not fully understood; researchers have only recently determined that measurable hormonal changes take place during a flash. Diminished estrogen levels are somehow responsible, but exactly in what way remains a bit unclear. Withdrawal of estrogen causes an increase in the levels of the hormones FSH and LH. The brain center that secretes these hormones, the hypothalamus, directs many body functions, including body temperature, sleep patterns, metabolic rate, mood, and reaction to stress. The higher the levels of FSH and LH, the more the blood vessels dilate, or enlarge, which increases blood flow to the skin, raising its temperature.

Levels of other hormones and body chemicals also seem to fluctuate in response to altered estrogen levels, and may participate in triggering a hot flash. Two neurotransmitters, epinephrine and norepinephrine, interact with the hypothalamus and help control dilation and contraction of blood vessels. The brain's natural mood controllers, the beta-endorphins, drop in response to lowered estrogen and progesterone levels, and may also be involved. Hormones do not operate in a vacuum. A rise or fall in any one creates a cascading interplay that can affect any number of bodily functions.

WHO WILL HAVE HOT FLASHES?

The fact that hot flashes are somehow related to changing estrogen levels is undisputed. A sharp drop in estrogen can lead to more severe symptoms. Women who have had their ovaries surgically removed report immediate and unpleasant hot flashes. Damage to these organs in other ways may also reduce hormonal output and increase the likelihood of hot flashes. Because smoking diminishes hormone production and inhibits circulation, smokers can expect to suffer more than nonsmokers.

A gradual decline in estrogen results in fewer flashes. Women with more body fat complain less than smaller, thinner women because they produce a type of estrogen that keeps their estrogen levels higher. The goal of nutritional support is to accomplish this without burdening the body with excess estrogen and excess weight. A nutrient-rich diet can provide an optimum environment that will support your organs and glands so they will make the correct amount of hormones needed during this transition.

Hot flashes do not appear to be universal. In the Japanese culture, for example, they are rarely mentioned, and there is no word that refers precisely to this menopausal sign.[1] Since the Japanese language makes extremely subtle distinctions about body states, the absence of such a word is significant. The Maya in Mexico don't report hot flashes either.[2] Several studies suggest this may be linked to diet. One common denominator among cultures in which menopausal symptoms are few or nonexistent is that the women consume higher levels of estrogen-containing foods. Even though their endocrine systems operate in the same way as those of Western women, the additional hormonal support from their diets minimizes or prevents symptoms.[3] Their positive outlook about growing older should also be considered as another possible factor.

TREATING HOT FLASHES NATURALLY

You don't have to be menopausal to experience a hot flash. Waves of heat may hit anyone, of any age, who engages in behavior that forces the temperature-regulating system to step up its activity. The following triggers may bring on a hot flash.

Triggers for Hot Flashes

hot weather, drinks, clothes
spicy foods
caffeine (coffee, tea, chocolate, colas)
exercise (especially if you are out of condition)
vigorous lovemaking
drugs of all kinds
alcohol
large meals
meals eaten too quickly
stress

Exercise

Treatments that stabilize the autonomic nervous system (which controls involuntary responses) may temper hot flashes. Regular moderate exercise decreases FSH and LH levels, reducing and possibly eliminating symptoms.[4] The hypothalamus regulates the menstrual cycle, body temperature, and the autonomic nervous system. During menopause, it becomes supersensitive to outside signals; exercise can stabilize it and help restore more normal hormonal levels.

A recent study of 79 menopausal women showed that moderate and even severe symptoms of hot flashes and sweating were reduced in both frequency and severity with exercise.[5] Of note to midlife women who would rather have a root canal than join a gym is that the women in this study exercised three to four hours a week—not an unreasonable commitment of time.

Exercise is considerably more effective, however, if it is begun well in advance of menopause. If your body is not conditioned, the unfamiliar activity may stimulate the very response you are trying to avoid. Keeping the body in good working order enables it to handle discomfort with greater ease. To minimize midlife and aging symptoms, increase your physical activity level.

Deep Breathing

Relaxation methods that consciously relax both the mind and the body have been shown to reduce hot flashes. In a pilot study of 33 postmenopausal women who reported having at least five hot flashes a day, it was found that slow, deep breathing alone reduced the incidence of hot flashes by about 50 percent.[6] Researchers concluded that women who are unable to receive hormone replacement therapy might benefit from this technique.

It makes sense. If stress is a trigger for flashes, then activities that can reduce the surge of hormones related to anxiety would be beneficial. Many books describe relaxation and deep-breathing techniques. My favorite is the classic by Herbert Benson, *The Relaxation Response*. If you can't wait to purchase the book and want to start immediately, here is a summary of the basic breathing technique. Sit in a comfortable position. Close your eyes and relax all your muscles. Slowly breathe in and out through your nose, becoming aware of each breath. It sounds easy, but distractions will continually infiltrate your thoughts, breaking the mood. Attempt to disregard these intrusions and to keep breathing deeply for 10 to 20 minutes.

Diet

Good dietary habits and additional nutritional support can often help in preventing and treating hot flashes. Hormones are formed from the building blocks of food, and if even one nutritional element is missing, a hormonal deficiency or imbalance may result. Preventing a physical ailment is always preferable to curing it, so nurturing the organs and glands with the right foods should be a primary goal throughout life.

Sweets and Treats

Reducing minimally nutritive foods is crucial for menopausal women. After-dinner sweets, specialty coffees, and dinner wines, as comforting as they are, do not serve menopausal women well. If you are already well into menopause, you may have noticed your favorite treats are not as well tolerated as they were a few years ago. The same coffee and chocolate at night that delighted you before may now keep you up until dawn with nightmares, a racing heartbeat, and hot flashes. Pay attention to foods that are no longer worth the momentary pleasure.

Overdosing on sweets is especially aggravating to the body at menopause. A high sugar intake stresses the adrenal gland and pancreas at a time when both need to be in good working order. London University's John Yudkin, in his book *Sweet and Dangerous*, warns against the ill effects refined sugar can have on the hormones. A high-sugar diet, he reports, "can cause a striking increase in the level of adrenal cortical hormone . . . . It can slow the rate of transport of hormonal chemical by as much as two thirds even in one week."[7] Sometimes just regulating your sugar intake may control uncomfortable hot flashes. Over the long term, high sugar intake may cumulatively weaken the adrenal glands so that estrogen is not converted efficiently. Remember, at menopause the adrenal glands take over the production of estrogen; when they can make this change smoothly, symptoms are less intense and infrequent.

Blood-sugar fluctuation, or *hypoglycemia*, is clearly a factor in the experience of hot flashes.[8] If your first sign of approaching menopause is a hot flash, stop and consider your diet. In fact, do more than think about it: write down what you eat for a week or two. This may strike you as unnecessary, but a recent poll by the Human Nutrition Research Center found that over 80 percent of the population either under- or overestimates their food intake. It appears few of us are clear about the calories, sugar, salt, fat, and nutrients we consume daily, and tracking our diet can be enlightening.

Phytohormones: The Latest Good News

There has been a lot of excitement in the women's health community in the last two years about two emerging natural treatments, phytohormones and natural progesterone. Before hormone replacement therapy was discovered, traditional cultures used certain foods and herbs to treat a range of female complaints. Research today confirms that many menopausal women who do not experience flashes have a plant-based or primarily vegetarian diet. We now know that some plants and common foods, herbs, and spices contain natural substances, called *phytohormones*, which help the body produce its own natural estrogen and progesterone. These phytohormones are also called *adaptogens* because they work within the system to balance hormonal levels—raising them if they are too low and lowering them if they are too high.

Phytohormones, also called phytosterols, are structurally and functionally similar to steroid hormones. While these plant hormones do not actually contain human hormones, they do encourage their production within the body. Because plant hormones act systemically, they treat a broad range of conditions, such as hot flashes and vaginal dryness, menstrual irregularities, and fibroid tumors. They appear to improve blood flow to female organs, keep arteries clear, and offer protection from cancer.

Plant hormones have a safety record centuries long. Compared with commercially prepared drugs, their potency is very low and they stimulate a woman's body to produce the hormones she needs without toxic side effects. Much like the body's natural secretions, phytohormones keep arterial pathways clear and help elevate the good HDLs (*high density lipoproteins*, the type of cholesterol that removes excessive cholesterol from the blood).[9] Unlike synthetic estrogen, phytoestrogens appear to have no down side. While the synthetic form carries with it the threat of breast cancer, plant-based estrogen effectively inhibits mammary tumors.[10]

Natural Sources of Phytohormones[13]

Alfalfa	Oats
Anise	Orchard grass
Apples	Palmetto grass
Barley	Parsley
Bluegrass	Peas
Carrots	Pomegranates
Cherries	Potatoes
Coffee	Rape seed
Date palms	Red beans
Fennel	Rice
French beans	Rye
Garlic	Sage
Green beans	Sesame
Hops	Soybeans
Licorice	Wheat

Phytohormones abound in nature. There are hundreds —perhaps even thousands— within the cells of plant foods we eat everyday. They have long been sipped in teas and tinctures to relieve a range of symptoms. And foods such as soybeans and yams form the basis of medicinal hormones used to treat menstrual as well as menopausal discomfort. Check the Resources section of this book for information on these products, and be aware that your physician may not know about natural alternatives.

Dietary phytosterol intake among populations differs dramatically. People who eat a vegetarian diet take in about 345 mg to 400 mg per day, compared to the 80 mg a day of people consuming a more Western diet.[11] Studies show they also suffer much less from hot flashes and other menopausal signs. So, there is a strong probability that if women were to incorporate more plant foods rich in natural hormones into their diets, hot flashes and other menopausal symptoms would lessen.

Clinical tests show the highest amount of these natural compounds are found in soy products, specifically tofu.[12] Tofu is made by adding a curdling agent to soymilk and then pressing the soybean curd into cubes. Tofu is becoming more popular in the United States and can be found in many markets. The beauty of tofu is its blandness: it takes on the flavor of the food or sauce in which it is prepared. It is extremely versatile and can replace meat in casseroles, chili, lasagna, or enchiladas. You can stir-fry it with vegetables, or add it to soups and stews. A great book of recipes for tofu and other soy products is *The Simple Soybean and Your Health* by Mark and Virginia Messina.

Consuming more grains, fruits, and vegetables—with special emphasis on those high in phytohormones—may take you through menopause more smoothly. Remember, natural remedies do take time; results may take three or four months.

Natural Progesterone

Plant hormones can also be synthesized in the laboratory to produce medicinal hormones. Progesterone, for example, can be extracted from the wild yam to provide a natural alternative to the hormone used in hormone replacement preparations. Researchers find natural progesterone is biochemically closer to the molecular structure of the progesterone found in the female body than is the synthetic compound used in hormone replacement therapy. Also, since it is absorbed through the skin, it bypasses liver metabolism. For this reason, it appears to be safer and shows none of the side effects so often associated with the synthetic hormone.

Wild yam progesterone comes as an over-the-counter cream or oil or can be prescribed in pill form by a physician. It is being used clinically to treat menopausal symptoms as well as a variety of female conditions. Some research suggests that natural estrogen and progesterone taken in pill form is as effective as the synthetic version, yet offers fewer side effects and less long-term risk. An excellent source of information on natural progesterone is *Natural Progesterone: The Multiple Roles of a Remarkable Hormone* by John Lee, M.D., who has pioneered its use in treatment.

Several brands of progesterone cream containing this natural progesterone are now available over-the-counter, such as Pro-Gest, Progonol, Ostaderm, and Progesterone. These creams can be found in health-food stores and pharmacies. They are generally applied to the skin twice a day in small amounts.

Nutrients That Suppress Hot Flashes

✦ **Vitamin E**   Clinical studies have shown certain nutrients to be effective in treating hot flashes. The most widely recommended is vitamin E. Medical journals first published studies of vitamin E as a treatment for hot flashes in the late 1940s. However, with the advent of estrogen therapy and tranquilizers, nutritional solutions were largely forgotten. More money could be made from a drug than an unpatentable natural product. Only when it became clear that not all women were safe candidates for hormonal therapy did researchers dust off their books to rediscover this already-proven alternative.

Early studies in the late 1940s tested women who could not be treated with estrogen because they had estrogen-based tumors. All the women suffered from unremitting hot flashes and mood changes. After taking vitamin E, the women experienced either complete relief or marked improvement—without side effects.[14] Other early studies confirmed this finding.

Vitamin E is a hormone normalizer. Tests indicate that when vitamin E is low, the levels of FSH and LH increase. Since these hormones already tend to be overabundant in menopausal women, a shortage of vitamin E could exacerbate the situation. Vitamin E appears to have a stabilizing effect on estrogen levels, increasing the hormone output in women who are deficient and lowering it in those who are prone to excess. Adequate doses can buffer the hormonal ebbs and flows during the change, relieving associated symptoms. Other menopausal symptoms that are helped by supplemental vitamin E include nervousness, fatigue, insomnia, dizziness, heart palpitations, shortness of breath, and vaginal dryness.[15]

Many nutritionists agree that the increase of refined foods in our diet, coupled with the absence of whole grains, nuts, and seeds, has led to a dangerous decline in dietary vitamin E. To compound the problem, vitamin E is destroyed when it is exposed to air or heated, frozen, or stored. While most of us experience minor short-ages of vitamin E that rarely degenerate into a classic "deficiency disease," the weakness engendered on the deeper, cellular level makes us susceptible to a host of symptoms, some of which appear to be directly related to menopause.

For relief of hot flashes, Barbara and Gideon Seaman recom-mend starting with 100 IU of vitamin E, and gradually increasing the dosage over a few weeks to a few months until you experience results.[16] It may take up to 1,200 IU daily before reduction in the frequency or intensity of the hot flashes is apparent.

Vitamin E should be complemented with the mineral sele-nium, as studies show that the two operate synergistically: their combined effect is greater than either taken alone.

Note: If you have high blood pressure, diabetes, or a rheu-matic heart condition, do *not* take more than 30 IU of vitamin E without first checking with your physician.

As a fat-soluble nutrient, vitamin E is absorbed from the intestinal tract only in the presence of fat. To ensure absorption, take vitamin E with a meal incorporating some fat—not, for exam-ple, with grapefruit and coffee. You can also aid its digestibility and utilization by taking it with lecithin, a fat that has been reported to reduce the incidence of hot flashes.

Good sources of vitamin E are the following: sunflower seeds, almonds, crab, sweet potatoes, fish, wheat germ, and whole wheat bread. For the precise amount of this nutrient contained in certain foods, consult Appendix C.

✦ Bioflavenoids   Bioflavenoids function as weak estrogens and can be taken with vitamin C to relieve hot flashes and vaginal dryness. Like vitamin E, these vitaminlike substances have been successfully used in cancer patients for whom estrogen replacement therapy is contraindicated. Dosages range from 500 mg to 2,000 mg per day, and they are absorbed better when taken in divided doses.

There are over 200 bioflavenoids, such as rutin, hesperidin, and quercetin; hesperidin is recommended by some as being especially useful for menopausal complaints. The best dietary sources are the white pulp beneath the peel of citrus fruits; the skin of grapes, cherries, and berries; leafy vegetables; and wine.

✦ **Herbal remedies**   In the mid-1800s, Lydia Pinkham concocted a vegetable compound to cure female maladies. For over 100 years, her company sold her natural potion as an alternative to medical prescriptions. Women have long passed down tried-and-true herbal remedies, but until recently, modern medicine held that these recipes merely provided a placebo effect for the "hysterical" woman. No longer. Herbs that were once considered worthless are now being studied for the treatment of many ailments.

Not surprisingly, the herbs found most effective for menopausal complaints are similar to those in Lydia Pinkham's original formula. These herbs, known to be natural sources of estrogenic substances, act on the pituitary and adrenal glands to stabilize the menstrual cycle. They include fenugreek, gotu kola, sarsaparilla, licorice root, and wild yam root. Nan Koehler, a botanist and herbalist, suggests making a tea with one of these herbs combined with another herb high in minerals, such as dandelion leaves, alfalfa, or borage.

✦ **Ginseng**   Ginseng, a popular and potent herb, has been studied for 5,000 years and millions of people the world over praise its stimulating qualities. In several countries it is used for temperature imbalances, such as chronic sweating, heat stress, and hot flashes. It, too, is said to exert a "normalizing" action on the pituitary gland, as well as to help in rebuilding tissues, stimulating energy, enhancing physical and mental performance, regulating blood pressure, reducing cholesterol, and generally rejuvenating the body, strengthening it against the debilitating effects of stress. Ginseng is also believed to increase estrogen levels and is recommended for women at menopause.

Ginseng is available in many forms, some more energizing than others. The primary active agents in ginseng, called *ginsenosides*, are found in different proportions depending on where and how the ginseng is grown. Some forms tend to stimulate the body; others relax and cool it.

Oriental cultivated ginseng, also called *panax*, is of the energy-producing variety and is commonly available in health food stores in capsules, extracts, and teas. Siberian ginseng, often labeled just ginseng, is not a true ginseng but it is a related plant with the same energy-enhancing properties. Studies show that the Siberian extract improves the performance of long-distance runners, demonstrating its strengthening and endurance-building properties. American ginseng offers more of the cooling properties and is better for regulating the temperature control system.

Unlike most vitamins, ginseng is most effective when taken on an empty stomach. Dosage varies, so follow the package directions. You can drop the capsules into hot water for a soothing tea. It is best not to take it with vitamin C or food high in vitamin C since ascorbic acid tends to neutralize it. None of the tests to which modern scientists have subjected this ancient herb have shown it to have a single deleterious side effect.[17]

✦ **Vitex (vitex agnus-castus)**   Vitex, also known as chaste tree or chasteberry, is regarded throughout Europe as *the* herb for menopause, PMS, and uterine fibroid cysts. It profoundly stimulates pituitary function, altering LH and FSH secretions. Using vitex regularly for a few months will increase your natural levels of progesterone and help control hot flashes, depression, and a dry vagina. One caution: it is not to be taken with birth control pills.

Like most herbs, vitex comes in many varieties. The bottles will provide the appropriate dosage, usually 1 capsule up to 3 times daily or 10 to 30 drops of extract in juice or water up to 3 times daily. For optimum benefit, take it for at least 3 months. Herbs and nutrients restore balance to the body slowly and gently.

Herbs can be taken individually or in concert with others. Black cohosh, sage, dong quai, wild yam, and sarsaparilla combine well with vitex. Some mixtures may be labeled as "menopausal formulas." Experiment until you find one that works for you.

WHERE DO I START?

If you are bothered by incessant hot flashes, start by eliminating foods that are obvious triggers. Check your diet to see if you are promoting blood-sugar extremes. Fasting all day and overindulging at night can be just as devastating to the body as gulping down four cups of coffee and two chocolate-filled croissants. Check that your diet contains adequate amounts of the nutrients mentioned. If not, add foods that incorporate these vitamins or supplement as indicated. When supplementing, try one nutrient or herb at a time so as not to overwhelm the body. If you have an allergic reaction, the source will be obvious.

Your body is unique, and your program will be individual as well. Just because vitamin E worked for your friend does not mean it will remedy your flashes. Dr. Atkins, author of *Dr. Atkins' Nutritional Breakthrough* and other books, describes the determined endeavors it takes to find the right natural remedy: "While vitamin E in 800 IU worked for one woman, another tried vitamin E, diet, ginseng, dong quai and still didn't feel better until lecithin was added to her regimen."[18]

Natural Remedies for Hot Flashes

✦ Exercise moderately and regularly.

✦ Use deep breathing or relaxation techniques.

✦ Eliminate triggers: sugar, coffee, alcohol, spicy foods, hot drinks, warm clothes.

✦ Maintain a constant blood-sugar level:
Eat every 4 to 5 hours.
Watch concentrated sugar, caffeine, and alcohol.
Don't overeat.

✦ Include one or more of the following in your daily diet:
vitamin E (800–1,200 IU, divided into 1 to 3 doses), mixed tocopherols preferred;
selenium (15–50 mcg);
lecithin (6–12 capsules, divided into 1 to 3 doses);
vitamin C with bioflavenoids (1,000–3,000 mg spread throughout the day);
herbs: ginseng, vitex, black cohosh, sage, sarsaparilla, licorice root, wild yam root, dong quai, yarrow.

4

FATIGUE

Female fatigue is the most common
"Silent Disease" of women.
—ELIZABETH WEISS, *FEMALE FATIGUE*

How often do you say that you feel tired and listless, that you lack energy at the end of the day? Such complaints come not only from menopausal women but from women of all ages. What is most exasperating is that, in the majority of cases, doctors report no physiological basis for these symptoms. Boredom, stress, depression, and psychosomatic tendencies are often suggested as explanations for fatigue. This may be accurate, but let's consider some equally valid possibilities.

Excessive fatigue during perimenopause is usually due to interruptions in sleep because of hot flashes or other disturbances triggered by hormonal irregularities. Lack of continuous restful sleep tends to wear one down both physically and emotionally. Once the hormones stabilize, sleep patterns and energy generally return to normal. If you feel the hours you spend sleeping are adequate, but the tiredness still lingers, look to other possibilities.

Energy levels depend on many factors, some psychological, some physiological. Three culprits stand out among the physiological causes of chronic fatigue: low blood sugar, anemia, and underactive thyroid. Each condition can be the result of several factors; the most likely but least considered are the nutritional ones. In other words, these conditions can often be created and treated by the foods we do or don't eat.

Remember, as our organs age, they lose resilience. Many foods we once devoured with relish gradually become toxic to our bodies. Our glandular system needs to be treated with greater respect with each passing birthday.

LOW BLOOD SUGAR

Almost all of us experience the late-morning or the mid-afternoon "droops" and regard it as a normal part of our daily routine. If we haven't eaten in several hours, it is not especially surprising that we feel tired and weak, have a headache, cannot think clearly, lose our temper, and crave sweets. We may be inclined to ignore these symptoms, but we should not. Our body is communicating something to us: we are being warned of a metabolic imbalance that, left unchecked, could lead to far greater problems.

The metabolic irregularity to which I refer is called hypoglycemia, or, more commonly, low blood sugar. Hypoglycemia results from an imbalance in the body's sugar-regulating mechanism that prevents the maintenance of a stable level of sugar in the blood. The body breaks down carbohydrates (starches and sugars) into glucose, the fuel with which we operate. If too much glucose is circulating in the body, the excess is taken out of the blood with the help of the hormone insulin and is stored in the liver as glycogen. As the fuel is used up in daily activity, glycogen is gradually converted back into glucose, thus maintaining a stable blood-sugar level.

When the system is flooded with sugar, this equilibrium is disrupted and the body goes into a tailspin. Nearly every organ and gland must work overtime in a furious attempt to bring the blood-sugar level back to normal. For a while we feel ready to take on the problems of the world, but the elation is short-lived. The pancreas, reacting to what it perceives as an emergency, pours extra insulin into the bloodstream, which withdraws the sugar from the blood and restores equilibrium. In its exuberance, the overcompensating pancreas usually withdraws too much sugar, causing the blood-sugar level to drop dangerously low. We now experience fatigue, weakness, shakiness, loss of coordination, headaches, hostility, and a craving for more sugar. To ease these unsettling feelings, to "calm our nerves," we grab a cookie, cola, cigarette, or cup of coffee. This may provide momentary relief, but the pancreas over-reacts again, the cycle continues, up and down, day after day, year after year. Ultimately, the glands and the organs weaken.

Sugar

Eating too much sugar is probably the greatest crime we women perpetrate against our bodies. When we are bored, anxious, happy, or depressed, we eat. Even women who restrain their urges three weeks a month may succumb two days before their periods and head straight for the nearest chocolate bar. It is not surprising that we suffer anxiety mixed with fatigue when we choose to subject our bodies to this roller-coaster existence.

Many men—especially the male-dominated medical estab-lishment—use an expression to explain the turbulent feelings sup-posedly experienced by women in connection with life transitions and menstrual events: "raging hormones." This absurd expression has been used to dismiss all female complaints. While our hor-mone levels do vary at different stages in our lives, whether or not they "rage" may relate to factors other than the female cycle. A blood-sugar imbalance resulting from stress or improper diet could easily cause a mood swing. And if that is so, men too can suffer from "raging hormones."

A woman may experience fatigue from a blood-sugar imbal-ance even if she is not a diagnosed hypoglycemic. Low blood sugar is relative; even if a person falls well within the normal range (60–120 mg) on a glucose tolerance test, she may experience symp-toms. Barbara Edelstein finds that when blood sugar drops suddenly, even though not to a critical level, some women get very anxious, some burst into tears, some feel shaky, and some become confused.[1]

Other conditions that can precipitate blood-sugar imbalances include severe and prolonged stress, pregnancy, lactation, cancer, tumors, chronic infection, and glandular malfunction. Be on the alert if any of these conditions describe you.

For the most part, hypoglycemia is self-induced. By persist-ently eating highly refined carbohydrates such as concentrated sug-ars and white bread, drinking endless cups of coffee, and smoking cigarettes, we upset the delicate blood-sugar mechanism. Years of abuse render many of the endocrine glands ineffective. As a result, the adrenal and pituitary glands, pancreas, and liver may all produce decreased amounts of hormones no matter how much they are stimulated. Eventually, even minor stresses (large helpings of cake or ice cream) turn into major events as the body, worn out from misuse, overreacts or refuses to respond.

The human biochemical system is not adapted to handle large amounts of concentrated sugar. Not only is refined sugar devoid of nutritional value, it leaches the body's vitamin and mineral reserves in the effort made to digest it. All carbohydrates require certain nutrients to be metabolized, the most important of which are the B-complex vitamins. Without adequate amounts of these vitamins, sugar ferments in the digestive tract and is converted to acetic acid and alcohol. Too much sugar coupled with too few B vitamins results in overacidity, gross nutritional imbalances, and low blood sugar.

I am not suggesting complete self-denial or a lifetime without chocolate cake. Realistically, if you can get by without sugar for five days out of seven you are doing very well; six days out of seven is excellent. Remember, the older your body is, the less able it is to bounce back from dietary indiscretions. Be good to yourself— decrease your sugar intake and increase your ratio of good to not-so-good days. On the days when you have that special treat, supplement with a B-complex vitamin. The ill effects will be reduced and symptoms may be more moderate.

Many of us who were brought up on dessert after every meal have a hard time believing that sugar is all that harmful. The facts, unfortunately, are clear. Refined carbohydrates in general, and refined sugar in particular, have been implicated in a wide array of health problems, from obesity, diabetes, coronary thrombosis, and tooth decay to high blood pressure, menstrual cramps, premenstrual syndrome, cancer, and mental disturbances. In countries where people live primarily on whole foods, many of these problems are absent. When refined sugar and refined carbohydrates are introduced to these countries, the "diseases of civilization" emerge within 10 years.

The constant need for sugar has been compared to addiction. William Dufty, a self-proclaimed former "sugar addict," writes in his book *Sugar Blues* that the only difference between a sugar habit and narcotic addiction is one of degree: "Sugar takes a little longer, from a matter of minutes in the case of a simple sugar like alcohol, to a matter of years in sugars of other kinds."[2] This may seem a bit of an exaggeration, but try going two days without your nightly raid on the refrigerator or your afternoon pick-me-up, and then think about it.

Your body is always giving you signals, telling you when something is not working correctly. Fatigue is only one of the warnings of an erratic blood-sugar level. If you have the symptoms listed below, be particularly cautious about the amount of concentrated sugar you consume, and if you feel you can't possibly give up sugar, I urge you to read Bill Dufty's book. His story of how he kicked his "habit" is fascinating, and his practical instructions for change are most helpful.

Symptoms of Low Blood Sugar

+ sudden feelings of nervousness, a sensation of "going crazy"

+ periods of irritability for no reason

+ spurts of energy after meals, followed by quick exhaustion

+ sudden feelings of faintness or dizziness

+ periodic bouts of depression

+ sudden headaches

+ temporary feelings of forgetfulness and confusion

+ unprovoked anxiety and worry

+ feelings of internal trembling

+ heart palpitations

+ rapid pulse not accompanying exercise

+ abnormally antisocial feelings

+ indecisiveness

+ crying spells

+ unexplained phobias

+ frequent nightmares

+ cravings for sweets

+ indigestion, gas, colitis

Diagnosing Low Blood Sugar

Hypoglycemia is a disease with many causes, including a number of genetic, functional, and dietary imbalances. Because it is known to imitate other disease states, a comprehensive examination and a six-hour glucose tolerance test are essential for identifying severe problems. It is best to look for a nutrition-oriented physician or nutritionist because many orthodox physicians are not trained to recognize nutritional imbalances. Richard Brennan, founder of the International Academy of Preventive Medicine, claims that "despite hypoglycemia's seriousness, nine out of ten physicians who come in contact with the disease misdiagnose it."[3] Most physicians do not treat the problem but treat the symptoms. Often, and I think this is especially true in the case of women, they dismiss the patient as a hypochondriac.

Clearly, in order to have a disease diagnosed and treated, you must see a medical doctor. The point I am making is that most physicians are not trained to recognize and treat nutritional problems, and there *are* problems caused by inappropriate nutrition. So, if your doctor is unable to find a functional disturbance and your symptoms persist, consider seeing a nutritionist.

Caffeine

Sugar is not the only factor to consider if your blood-sugar level is erratic. Coffee, chocolate, cola, and certain teas contain caffeine, which plays havoc with the body's sugar mechanism. Caffeine stimulates the adrenal cortex to produce more adrenalin, which in turn induces the liver to break down glycogen into glucose. Many people are unaware that caffeine is hidden in many soft drinks and in common over-the-counter medications such as Anacin, Excedrin, Midol, and appetite suppressants.

Alcohol

Alcohol is a central nervous depressant, so drinking too much can increase fatigue and exacerbate depression. It can intensify hot flashes and insomnia, so menopausal women who are already experiencing these symptoms might control the wine with dinner for a while. Physicians who have studied alcoholism believe that hypoglycemia may be a prime causative factor in this addiction.[4]

Cigarettes

Cigarettes change the rate at which the body handles food. A clinical experiment found that women who smoke more than 15 cigarettes a day are apt to be fatigued as a result of the amount of nicotine their bodies are required to metabolize. Although the harmful effects of smoking can be partly offset through nutrient supplements, it is far better to end the habit. In preparation for quitting smoking, you can fortify your body by taking the following daily: a high-potency multiple vitamin and mineral tablet; vitamin C, 1,000–3,000 mg; vitamin E, 400–1,000 IU (dry form); selenium, 50 mcg 1 to 3 times; and cysteine, 500–1,000 mg. In addition, take vitamin A, 10,000 IU, daily for five days, then stop for two.[5] A great book that explains how nicotine and other ingredients in cigarettes affect women's bodies is *How Women Can* Finally *Stop Smoking* by Dr. Robert Klesges and Margaret DeBon.

Stress

Stress in any form—physical, emotional, chemical, or nutritional—overworks the adrenal glands and can bring about blood-sugar imbalances. Since we cannot avoid all emotional stressors, and often cannot escape environmental chemical stresses, we should learn to deal with those conditions over which we *do* have control: the physical and nutritional factors. We can physically strengthen our bodies through exercise and nourish them with food and supplements, tipping the balance in favor of regeneration rather than degeneration. And let's not underestimate the recuperative power of meditation and relaxation therapy, biofeedback, water immersion, and massage.

DIETARY RECOMMENDATIONS FOR CONTROLLING BLOOD SUGAR

Blood-sugar imbalances can be controlled through a dietary program that reestablishes biochemical balance. Since many factors can raise or lower the blood-sugar level, it is important to treat the whole person. Minor imbalances can be controlled through diet, but in extreme situations heavy nutrient supplements may be needed.

To reverse high blood-sugar levels and to relieve fatigue, your diet must be designed for a slow release of insulin from the pancreas, ensuring a steady release of glucose into the blood throughout the day. The foods to emphasize for such a program are protein (meat, fish, cheese, tofu, seeds, and nuts) and complex carbohydrates (vegetables, beans, whole grain breads and cereals, and some fruits). A small percentage of people with volatile blood-sugar regulatory problems may have to limit their intake of carbohydrates; they seem to operate best by emphasizing primarily protein-rich foods. Experiment and see what works best for you.

Smaller, more frequent meals are recommended, as well as the elimination of concentrated sugars (even fruit juice, for sensitive people), caffeine, cigarettes, marijuana, and certain medications. A long list of prescription drugs can play havoc with your blood-sugar levels and may create puzzling symptoms. Some medications that may send your sugar levels in either direction are anabolic steroids, estrogen, cortisone, lithium, thiazide, barbiturates, sulfonamides, and beta blockers. Ask your doctor about your prescriptions, if you have any.

Exercise improves blood sugar regulation and the receptivity of the cells to insulin. It is a great hormone normalizer and does wonders for raising your spirits and increasing your energy.

Supplemental Program

Eating properly may not be enough for a person with a severe imbalance. Physicians who treat hypoglycemia find that between-meal nutrient supplements must be included. People whose diets have been deficient for years in vitamins and minerals, amino acids, and unsaturated fatty acids require greater than standard amounts of these nutrients to reverse the negative hypoglycemic cycle.[6]

✦ **B vitamins** The inability to handle stress and an uncontrolled desire for sugar are major factors in the development of hypoglycemia. Both conditions quickly burn B vitamins, leaving the body devoid of energy. A B-complex vitamin supplement can compensate for this deficiency. I recommend a formula that contains 20–30 mg each of vitamins B-1, B-2, B-3, and B-6, and 100–500 mg of pantothenic acid. Food sources rich in B vitamins include desiccated liver, wheat germ, peas, beans, and brewer's yeast. The B vitamins generally occur in the same foods, so a deficiency of one usually indicates a deficiency of the others.

✦ **Vitamin A** A variety of nutrients participates directly and indirectly in maintaining blood-sugar balance. Without the complete array of these nutrients, glandular functions are diminished and hormonal output becomes erratic. For example, hormones from the adrenal cortex are very sensitive to a vitamin A deficiency. If adequate vitamin A is not available, cortisone, the adrenal hormone that balances the effects of insulin, will not be synthesized.

You may be eating foods with vitamin A and still be deficient. While carotenes, which are food pigments that convert to vitamin A, occur in large amounts in green and yellow vegetables, many people have difficulty converting these into the usable nutrient. Carotenes come in many forms; beta carotene is the most important and most common. If you have difficulty converting carotene to vitamin A, you may need supplements. An appropriate range for most adults is 5,000 to 20,000 IU. Good sources of vitamin A are the following: liver, crab, carrots, sweet potatoes, pumpkin, spinach, broccoli, and cantaloupe. For the precise amount of this nutrient contained in certain foods, consult Appendix C.

✦ **Vitamin C** Vitamin C is also important in the utilization of sugar. In 1977, Fred Dice of Stanford University reported that the dose of insulin required to control the sugar level in a diabetic who lacked the ability to produce the hormone was cut in half when the patient took high doses of vitamin C.[7]

The ability of vitamin C to produce energy and reduce fatigue has been noted by many scientists. It is thought that vitamin C cleanses the body of pollutants and blocks the formation of carcinogens found in foods and in the body. It also may prevent "tired blood" (blood that is low in oxygen, thereby slowing down its energy-producing functions) by increasing the production of leukocytes (white blood cells that fight infection) and hemoglobin (red blood cells that carry oxygen to all the cells). Without this important vitamin, energy-giving iron would be ineffective. In one study, over 400 people were interviewed; those who took more than 400 mg of vitamin C per day clearly experienced less fatigue than people who were not supplementing.[8] Good sources of vitamin C are the following: orange juice, broccoli, brussels sprouts, grapefruit juice, strawberries, and raw tomato. For the precise amount of this nutrient contained in certain foods, consult Appendix C.

✦ **Minerals**   The minerals magnesium, potassium, and chromium are all involved in the metabolization of carbohydrates and thus affect energy levels. Magnesium sparks more chemical reactions in the body than any other mineral, and an undersupply of magnesium can cause fatigue, weakness, and irritability. Most women do not take in enough of this mineral, which may partially explain pervasive complaints of fatigue. Good sources of magnesium are the following: peanuts, lentils, split peas, tofu, wild rice, bean sprouts, almonds, chicken, spinach, and beef.

Daily Supplements That Aid in Balancing Blood Sugar

multiple vitamin and mineral supplement

B-complex vitamins (20–30 mg), 3 times daily for extreme cases

pantothenic acid (100–500 mg)

vitamin A (5,000–10,000 IU)

vitamin C (50–500 mg)

magnesium (500 mg)

potassium (2,000–3,000 mg)

chromium (200 mcg)

Potassium deficiency can cause symptoms similar to those of low blood sugar. This was brought to public attention when American astronauts made one of their first lunar flights: they suffered heartbeat irregularities because the synthetic orange juice they drank lacked potassium. Excessive use of laxatives and diuretics, vomiting, diarrhea, or chronic low intake of water can lead to dehydration and possibly potassium deficiency symptoms. An adult typically ingests 1,875 to 5,625 mg daily. The recommended dosage for healthy people is 2,000 to 3,000 mg per day. Good sources of potassium are the following: fish, potatoes, avocado, bananas, nonfat milk, fresh peas, and oranges. For the precise amount of this nutrient contained in certain foods, consult Appendix C.

Chromium, too, is indispensable to the production of insulin and to metabolization of glucose. Chromium is best taken in a brewer's yeast product that contains the chromium compound called glucose tolerance factor (GTF), because this form is more easily absorbed and is better at stabilizing blood sugar than a standard chromium supplement. Studies show that 200 mcg daily significantly improve glucose tolerance.[9] Julian Whitaker, M.D., author of *Medical Secrets Your Doctor Won't Tell You*, routinely prescribes magnesium and potassium as he feels they are essential for good health, energy, and can be protective against heart disease, high blood pressure, and diabetes. He prefers a supplement of magnesium and potassium complexes with aspartate, an amino acid.[10]

Most Americans take in roughly 30 mcg of chromium daily, while the recommended range is 50 to 200 mcg. As with many minerals, absorption gradually deteriorates with age. Good sources of chromium are the following: all-bran cereal, puffed rice, orange juice, and cheese.

ANEMIA

Anemia is a reduction of the amount of hemoglobin in the blood or a reduction in the number of red blood cells. In either case, the reduced amount of oxygen available to the body cells causes decreased efficiency of body processes. The brain reacts to the lack of oxygen, causing headaches, dizziness, faintness, loss of memory, nervousness, irritability, and drowsiness. Other danger signs are rapid heartbeat, numbness and tingling in the fingers and toes, ringing in the ears, black spots in front of the eyes, and a craving for ice, dirt, clay, or laundry starch.

Anemia is never a disease in itself, but is always caused by other factors. The change in red blood cells may be due to the use of certain drugs, exposure to certain insecticides, infection or disease, endocrine disturbances, or bone marrow atrophy. Usually, however, anemia results from either chronic blood loss or a lack of adequate nutrients, most notably iron.

Iron

Since more than half the body's iron is present in the red blood cells as a component of hemoglobin, any blood loss results in iron depletion. Hemoglobin, the protein that transports oxygen from the lungs to the tissues and cells, not only houses the iron, but depends on it for its production. Even hemorrhoids or ulcers can cause enough blood loss to deplete iron stores. Anyone who continually loses blood obviously requires more iron.

During her childbearing years, a woman's requirement for iron is greater than a man's because she loses blood each month. If she has profuse or prolonged periods, or if she is using an intrauterine device (IUD), chances are she may be losing considerably more iron than is safe. IUD users are apt to develop iron deficiency because they lose up to five times the amount of blood other women do during menstruation.[11]

Inadequate iron in the blood is a pervasive problem in both young and middle-age women. Many studies reveal that the vast majority of women take in only one third to one half their total daily requirement. The reasons for this are twofold: they are not consuming enough iron-rich foods, and the iron in the foods they are eating is not being utilized completely by the body.

It is difficult to eat adequate amounts of iron-rich foods. Unless you love liver and can handle several cups of beans a day, you are unlikely to make the 18 mg RDA (recommended daily allowance) through diet alone. To combine foods high in iron is possible; unfortunately, not only would it require time and careful planning, but the amount of food needed would exceed 3,000 calories daily. Even if you did make the effort to eat the required amount of iron-rich foods each day, you would still have to take into account the fact that iron is poorly absorbed by the body. Lack of adequate stomach acid makes it difficult for many postmenopausal women to absorb iron. According to most sources, only 10 percent of the iron ingested is used by the body.

Good sources of iron are the following: liver, ground beef, dried apricots, blackstrap molasses, raisins, beans, cooked spinach, and chicken. For the precise amount of this nutrient contained in certain foods, consult Appendix C. For those who want to try to take care of their need for iron through diet alone, I offer some advice. When it comes to absorption, the best source of iron is liver. The other sources (spinach, peanut butter, legumes, nuts, wheat germ, molasses, apricots, and raisins) need nutritional assistance to do the job. James Cook, director of hematology at the University of Kansas Medical Center, suggests that if you combine grains, vegetables, and dried fruits with vitamin C, you can increase iron utilization as much as fourfold.[12]

Certain chemicals found in foods diminish the absorption of iron. Tannic acid (found in many teas), phytic acids (an ingredient in grains and cereals), and phosphates (a preservative added to most packaged bakery products, ice cream, and soft drinks) greatly decrease iron utilization.

Iron is lost through body excretions, such as sweat. If you exercise frequently, you may lose significant amounts of iron, so make sure your diet is generous in iron or take supplements.

A variety of iron supplements is available. Liver extracts provide the best meat source, called heme iron. Take tablets with meals. An absorbable form of nonheme or nonmeat iron includes iron bound to succinate, fumerate, ascorbate, glycinate, or apartate. These are better taken between meals, but if they cause abdominal discomfort, double the dose and take with meals.

Vitamin C aids in the absorption of iron and other minerals (especially calcium, copper, cobalt, and manganese). For optimum effect, take it with your iron-rich foods or supplement. If you are eating a well-balanced diet or take a multiple vitamin and mineral tablet, you are already getting sufficient amounts of these "micronutrients."

Folic Acid and B-12

Anemia and fatigue can be caused by a deficiency in nutrients other than iron. Lack of either folic acid (a vitamin found in both vegetable and animal sources) or vitamin B-12 may produce fatigue, as well as symptoms such as apathy, withdrawal, and slowed mental ability. Like iron, folic acid is involved in creating normal red blood cells. A deficiency causes fewer cells to be produced, which means less hemoglobin and eventually less oxygen to all the cells. Folic acid deficiency is common in women, especially in women taking or making excess estrogen, pregnant women, alcoholics, and the elderly. Folic acid and vitamin B-12 interconnect biochemically and are best taken together. Again, a good multiple vitamin tablet will include the full range of B vitamins.

UNDERACTIVE THYROID

Consider one more condition that can cause chronic fatigue before, during, or after menopause. Hypothyroidism, or an underactive thyroid, means that the gland is producing smaller than normal amounts of thyroid hormone. This condition may be widespread, yet frequently remains undetected. One does not need to wait until symptoms reach dramatic proportions; early, subtle complaints may be clues enough: fatigue, susceptibility to infection and disease, menstrual disorders, low body metabolism, unexplained weight gain, sensitivity to cold, constipation, loss of hair, dry skin, puffy eyes, and cold hands and feet. Obviously, these general indications could represent a number of problems. If you suspect they apply to you, follow up with self-help tests and, if indicated, check with your physician.

The symptoms of hypothyroidism are similar to those of hypoglycemia. According to Broda Barnes, a well-respected doctor who has published more than a hundred papers on the thyroid gland, there is a direct correlation between an underactive thyroid and blood-sugar imbalances; in fact, a drop in blood sugar is one of the symptoms of hypothyroidism.[13] As Barnes explains, when the thyroid is underactive, the liver is unable to release its stored glycogen and produce glucose, thereby causing a low blood-sugar condition. This theory has been tested in the laboratory: when the livers of laboratory animals are removed, blood sugar declines rapidly, and death from hypoglycemia occurs unless glucose is injected intravenously.

Self-Help Tests for Underactive Thyroid and Low Blood Sugar

Broda Barnes suggests that both hypoglycemia and hypothyroidism can be diagnosed at home. For hypoglycemia, simple observation of symptoms is sufficient. To detect an underactive thyroid, take your basal body temperature (the temperature of the body at rest) before arising in the morning. If it reads below 97.8 degrees, there is reason to suspect a thyroid deficiency. Repeat for three or four days to be certain of your reading. (For accurate basal temperature measurement, place a thermometer at your bedside. As you are awakening, place the thermometer in your armpit and keep it secure for 10 minutes. Menstruating women note: take your temperature the week of your period, since temperature is more subject to fluctuation during the remainder of the month.)

Iodine

The manufacturing of thyroid hormone is dependent on several nutrients, and the mineral iodine is at the top of the list. Deficiency of or an inability to metabolize iodine results in an enlargement of the gland, a condition known as *goiter*. A sore neck sometimes indicates a possible glandular dysfunction.

The most important dietary source of iodine is iodized salt (70 mcg of iodine per gram of salt). If you use iodized salt in cooking or sprinkle it on your food, there is little chance you need more. However, if your salt is not iodized, if you use sea salt, or if you are restricting your salt intake, you run the risk of being deficient.

Iodine cannot be presumed to be present in a "normal" diet. For example, while the daily requirement of 150 mcg can be easily obtained by eating saltwater fish or seaweed, one would have to eat 2 pounds of eggs, 6 pounds of meat, 8 pounds of cereal or nuts, or 10 pounds of vegetables or fruit to reach this amount.[14] If you are not a fish lover, consider supplementing your diet with kelp tablets. One tablet four times a day will stimulate production of the thyroid hormone in most individuals. Vitamin A and the mineral zinc must be present for iodine metabolization.

Selenium and Zinc

For the synthesis and metabolization of thyroid hormone, numerous nutrients and enzymes must work in concert. The importance of iodine is well-established. The effects of selenium deficiency on thyroid hormone concentration are not as profound as those of iodine deficiency; however, a lack of both selenium and zinc leads to severe hypothyroidism and goiter in rats.[15]

Vitamin B-1

Lack of vitamin B-1 (thiamine) will eventually slow thyroid function, and many of our everyday habits encourage this deficiency. Eating too much sugar is a primary cause of thiamine deficiency. The higher the sugar intake, the quicker and more intense the symptoms. Alcohol, coffee, and tobacco likewise eat up thiamine, creating what we commonly call a "hangover," "coffee nerves," or a "nicotine fit." Everyday stress, including the stress of exercise, increases thiamine demand, so joggers, dancers, and aerobics addicts, beware.

EXERCISE

When you are fatigued, the thought furthest from your mind is exercise, right? Right—and wrong. Try to overcome the urge to collapse; get out and do something. A brisk walk will stimulate your circulatory system and raise your metabolism. It might be a lack of physical activity that weakened your body's muscles and endocrine system in the first place. Oxygen is primary to every physical event in the body; a diminished supply results in a total degenerative effect. Exercise can combat fatigue and increase your energy and endurance by forcing oxygen to your brain, heart, digestive system, and throughout your body.

SETTING REALISTIC GOALS

One last comment concerning fatigue: don't overlook the obvious. You may be overtired because you are trying to do too much, trying to be everything to everybody, and running yourself ragged.

Examine your daily routine and responsibilities; maybe your lack of energy is caused by an impossible schedule. A good source for more information about the so-called superwoman syndrome is Georgia Witkin-Lanoil's *The Female Stress Syndrome: How to Recognize and Live with It*.[16] Remember, workaholism is also an addiction—and a disease.

HERBS FOR FIGHTING FATIGUE

Ginkgo biloba

Ginkgo biloba increases the flow of blood to the brain, improves memory, and has been successful in treating problems related to poor circulation. Recently it has been shown to increase the uptake of glucose by brain cells and improve the transmission of nerve signals.[17] An extract of the fresh leaves is marketed in the United States and Europe; the product should be standardized to contain 24 percent ginkgo flavonglycosides.

Ginkgo biloba is said to be the world's oldest surviving species, and can be traced back 200 million years. It has been cultivated in China as a sacred tree, and now it is grown widely across the United States. Ginkgo leaves have been used in Chinese medicine for their beneficial effect on the brain. To increase your energy, take the standard dosage of 40 mg, 3 times a day. Pills are also available; take as recommended by the manufacturer.

Ginseng

For fatigue, take capsules of powdered Siberian ginseng in doses of 200 mg to 1,000 mg, 3 times a day for one to three months. It is better to use lower doses for a longer time than higher doses for a shorter time. Herbs work at the cellular level, and their tonic effect is not dramatic. Expect to wait a few weeks before noticing results. If you are having difficulties sleeping, do not take ginseng close to bedtime.

5

Sexual Changes

With all the complexity, with all the
difficulties, most midlife women will say,
"Sex? It's gotten better and better."

—LILLIAN B. RUBIN, *WOMEN OF A CERTAIN AGE*

Menopause does not mean the end of sex. Quite the contrary; for many women, the midlife years are especially sexually satisfying and creative. Think about it: after nearly 40 years, you are free from the fear of pregnancy and the bother of birth control devices, tampons, and pads. Better yet, opportunities that were few and far between when the kids were running in and out of the house are now available. An entire Saturday afternoon can be spent in a leisurely romantic interlude. You don't have to worry or hurry. Look forward to these days—they should be days of celebration.

More good news: some of the hormonal alterations women experience at menopause actually heighten their sexual response; for many women, sex is even more satisfying at 50 than at 20. People who think that women change into asexual beings at menopause should consider these revealing statements from *The Hite Report*[1]:

"I believe sexual desire increases with age. Enjoyment certainly increases—I can vouch for that."

"I didn't know getting older would make sex better! I'm 51 now and just getting started."

"I thought that menopause was the leading factor in my dry
and irritable vaginal tract. My doctors thought that it was
lack of hormones ... but with my new lover, I am reborn.
Plenty of lubrication, no irritation."

Why do we expect the sexual charge to abandon us once we
reach a certain age? I believe we are conditioned to expect this.
All through life we are subtly—and not so subtly—indoctrinated
by the media to believe that sex and beauty accompany youth.
The ads in popular magazines and on TV confirm this. So it is not
surprising that many older women, when they see a few lines on
their faces and feel a few extra pounds on their figures, feel less
desirable.

The emotional impact of these changes can be devastating
for some women. Kaylan Pickford observes that if a woman accepts
the idea that only in youth is there beauty, sexuality, and therefore
love, she falls into the trap of making unrealistic comparisons and
becomes insecure. To compare the first spring flower with a late
summer sunset is absurd. Pickford says that youth, middle age, and
old age should never be compared. They are each as unique and
beautiful as the changing seasons—each offers a fresh perspective,
a different experience.

SEX: IS IT ALL IN YOUR HEAD?

"A woman's sex life after menopause is determined more by her
psychological outlook than her physical changes," says John
Moran, gynecologist and director of the Well Woman Centre in
London. The fate of the libido seems to depend on a number of
factors, such as genetic makeup, early childhood upbringing, and
life experiences, all of which come into play long before menopause. Psychiatrists agree that the sex drive is predominantly psychological, though controlled to a degree by the amount of steroids
circulating in the blood. It is possible that women who complain
they do not "feel sexy" after the change did not feel that way
before menopause. An extensive Kinsey study found that some
women use menopause as an excuse to curtail sexual relationships
they were unenthusiastic about anyway.

To a large extent, however, how a woman responds sexually depends on the interest and response of her partner. Your husband or lover may be going through his or her own midlife crisis. While middle-age men do not experience the range of hormonal changes women do, they do undergo anatomical changes that can reduce their sexual responsiveness. Like the woman's ovaries, the man's testicles decrease in size. The *vas deferens,* the narrow tube that transports sperm, becomes narrower, and the sperm become thinner and less plentiful. It generally takes longer for the middle-age male to reach arousal and orgasm. If the man is unaware that this is normal, he may become overanxious, and he may transfer his insecurity to his partner. Researchers note that some women's psychological problems with sex during this time may be caused by men who, bewildered by their own changes in sexual performance, shift the blame to their partners.[2]

Around the half-century mark, both men and women confront new problems and must make adjustments. They sometimes switch jobs, realizing that if they intend to make a career change it had better be soon. Children entering college may become a financial burden. Illnesses may result in physical adjustments, economic insecurity, and emotional stress. The uncertainty arising from all these changes may be more responsible for sexual and marital problems than either hormonal or physiological changes.

It is said that the most difficult part of aging sexually is accepting it. Men and women need to realize that our physical responses inevitably slow down. This has nothing to do with our femininity or masculinity—it is normal. Allowing more time for sexual expression is important. The term *communication* may be overused, but maybe that is because talking honestly about your troubles is good, commonsense practice. Share what is happening in your body with your partner; together you can creatively pursue ways of finding mutual satisfaction.

Myths and misconceptions have defined sexual roles for too long. For modern adult women, it is time to differentiate between the facts and the fiction about aging, menopause, and sexual satisfaction. Correct information is the best ally we have in preparing for the change—or any change, for that matter.

PHYSICAL CHANGES

Women going through menopause experience physiological changes in their female organs and hormonal secretions, some of which may result in a temporary decline in their sexual responsiveness. As Dr. Moran explained to me, "The dramatic change in hormone levels during the menopause accounts for a variety of unpleasant symptoms; chiefly, tiredness, lack of energy, low self-esteem, and poor memory. If the common vasomotor symptoms— hot flashes, headaches, and night sweats—are present, these can also lead to a feeling of being unwell. With all these symptoms, it is not surprising that sexual pleasure is diminished."

In a study collecting data from a group of perimenopausal women, it was found that there was a close association with the number of hot flashes and the frequency of intercourse.[3] Women experiencing hot flashes had a lower level of sexual activity. This observation can be interpreted in two ways: women who have hot flashes do not want sex more regularly, or regular sexual activity is protective against hot flashes. Both are possible.

Losing sleep and feeling overtired are reasons enough for anyone, at any age, to lose interest in sex. The cessation of menstrual periods and declining levels of female hormones, however, do not in themselves affect sexual desire. In fact, there is increasing evidence that women's sexual interest and enjoyment do not decrease at midlife, but increase. This is because of the change in the ratio of male to female hormones. What few women realize is that the hormone most responsible for sexual arousal is the male hormone, testosterone. Although testosterone is present in the female system prior to menopause, its effect is tempered by the larger proportions of estrogen and progesterone. As these female hormones decrease at menopause, the proportion of testosterone increases. Indeed, there is increasing evidence that women's sexual interest and enjoyment do not fall at midlife, but rise because of the change in the ratio of male to female hormones.

Declining female hormone levels may not directly affect sexual response, but they do subtly alter the reproductive tissues, often leading to uncomfortable and even painful intercourse. The changes are most evident in the vagina, which becomes smaller, shorter, thinner, smoother, drier, and less elastic. As estrogen levels decline, blood flow to the genitals diminishes and secretions of vaginal mucus dwindle. A woman generally is slower to lubricate in response to sexual arousal and often takes a little longer to achieve orgasm, although, according to Niels Lauersen, gynecologist and professor of obstetrics at Mt. Sinai Hospital in New York City, the difference is not great—between seconds and minutes.[4] In any case, women need not feel insecure if they take longer to lubricate; remember that it also takes longer for the mature man to achieve erection. Actually, this is probably the first time in the sexual relationship in which arousal time is close to equal—for men and women close in age, that is.

Other parts of the female anatomy undergo minor changes. The cervix, ovaries, and uterus diminish in size; the *labia majora* (outer lips of the vagina) become thinner, paler, and smaller; the breasts lose some of their fat, firmness, and shape, and may even become slightly less sensitive; and clitoral stimulation may become irritating due to lack of lubrication. Some of these changes may be unnoticeable, while others may be annoying, but they are all normal.

NATURAL REMEDIES
FOR VAGINAL DRYNESS

In a few women, decreased elasticity of the vagina, along with the reduced ability to lubricate, may cause vaginal dryness so severe that intercourse becomes uncomfortable or painful. In severe cases, it may even cause bleeding. The usual medical treatment is estrogen replacement therapy (ERT). However, if estrogen is contraindicated for you or you would rather not take hormones, internal as well as external lubricants are available.

Dietary Aids

Phytoestrogens may provide natural internal lubrication by improving blood flow to uterine tissue. Plants such as soybeans and herbs such as ginseng that work within the enzyme system as adaptogens can stimulate a woman's body to produce additional estrogen—but only if she needs it.[5]

Of all foods, tofu, or soybean curd, contains the greatest amounts of *isoflavones* (phytohormones with estrogenlike properties).[6] (See Chapter 3 for more discussion of adaptogens.) Soy is now widely available in the United States in many forms. You can experiment with recipes by substituting soybeans for beans in soups, stews, and casseroles. Soy flour can replace wheat flour in breads, rolls, pancakes, and muffins. Vegetarians are familiar with soy-based alternatives to meat. If you have not sampled veggie burgers, frozen soy desserts, and soy cheese, I highly recommend them. And even your favorite latte or cappuccino (decaf, of course) can be made with soy milk.

Essential fatty acids help keep all the tissues of the body, including the skin, hair, and genital tissues, well lubricated internally. In our concern to limit the fats in our diets, we may go overboard and eliminate necessary EFAs (essential fatty acids). Two oils are classified as "essential" because the body cannot manufacture them; they must come from the diet. Linoleic acid, an omega-6 fatty acid, is primarily found in nuts and in seeds like flax, pumpkin, sesame, and sunflower seeds. The oils derived from these sources are good choices for salads and for taking as a supplement (about 1 to 2 tablespoons per day). Linolenic acid, of the omega-3 family, is primarily found in oils of fish like salmon, trout, and mackerel. If you would rather not rely on your diet for EFAs, there are many capsule supplements of essential oils that will help to internally moisturize your tissues. Try evening primrose oil, flaxseed oil, black currant seed oil, and borage oil. The typical dosage is 2 to 8 capsules per day. Diabetics should not take supplemental fish oils, but can eat cold water fish such as salmon, tuna, trout, herring, and sardines.

Women bothered by vaginal dryness need to avoid substances that will further sap moisture from the membranes, including alcohol, caffeine, diuretics, and antihistamines. They should also keep the body well hydrated by drinking 1 to 2 quarts of water each day.

Daily Nutritional Support for Female Tissues

NUTRIENT	AMOUNT
Vitamin A (beta carotene)	5,000–30,000 IU
Vitamin C	500–5,000 mg
Bioflavenoids	500–2,000 mg
Vitamin E	400–1,200 IU

For the precise amount of these nutrients contained in certain foods, consult Appendix C.

Specific **vitamins** support and maintain the health of the vaginal and urinary tissues. Without them, these organs atrophy and dry out.

Note: If you have high blood pressure, diabetes, or a rheumatic heart condition, do not take more than 30 IU of vitamin E without first consulting with your physician.

Herbs

The herb chaste tree (vitex) contains flavenoids, glycosides, and micronutrients that enhance hormonal production and revitalize vaginal tissues. Dosage is generally 1 capsule up to 3 times a day, taken on an empty stomach, or 20 drops of tincture 1 or 2 times a day. Motherwort and dong quai may also stimulate vaginal lubrication and your sex life.

External Lubricants

Vegetable oils can help moisturize the vagina, increasing sexual enjoyment. The most popular choice is vitamin E oil in liquid or suppository form, though most unscented massage oils will also work. Oil-based products such as petroleum jelly and baby oil should not be used since they tend to coat the vaginal lining and inhibit one's own natural secretions. In this age of AIDS, it is important to know that petroleum-based products weaken and break down latex condoms—another reason to avoid them. Water-based products plump up the vaginal tissue by providing additional moisture. Everyone is familiar with the old standby, K-Y Jelly, but there are new names on the market, such as Astroglide, Sensell, Probe, and Calendula cream.

For women who do not want to bother with lubricating just prior to intercourse, there is a moisturizer gel called Replens that lasts up to three days. It is inserted as a suppository and has the additional benefit of protecting against vaginal infection.

Natural progesterone creams, discussed in Chapter 3, are also recommended. John Lee started using natural progesterone for menopausal women who could not take estrogen and found that, in many cases, it not only reversed osteoporosis but reduced vaginal atrophying.[7]

NATURAL REMEDIES
FOR BLADDER INFECTIONS

Fifteen percent of menopausal women experience recurrent bladder infections. Typical symptoms are frequent and painful urination, increased nighttime urination, feeling a need to urinate even when the bladder is empty, pain in the lower abdomen, and strong or unpleasant smell to the urine. Infections sometimes get out of control and require medical attention. If this is the case, see a doctor. Frequent urination itself could indicate a diabetic condition. It is important to determine when it is appropriate to use natural methods and when professional services are necessary.

The primary goal in treating bladder infections naturally is to (1) enhance the normal environmental condition within the bladder (to encourage friendly bacterial growth), and (2) prevent harmful bacteria from invading and propagating within the urinary tract.

A woman's urethra is considerably shorter than a man's, and she is more susceptible to bacterial infections throughout her life. A few commonsense precautions can ward off a pesky problem.

Commonsense Advice for
Preventing Urinary Infections

+ Do not delay emptying your bladder, and always empty it completely. Retaining urine any length of time will increase your risk of infection.

+ Always empty your bladder immediately after sexual contact to keep unfriendly microbes from entering the urethra.

+ Avoid tight clothes—jeans, underwear, or pantyhose—and wear cotton-crotch underwear to keep the vaginal area as dry as possible; bacteria multiply in a warm, moist environment.

+ Hygiene sprays, bubble baths, and soaps may cause further irritation; if you suspect an infection, discontinue their use.

+ Take hot baths to relieve the pain associated with infection. Add one cup of vinegar to a shallow bath, and sit in it with your knees up so that water can enter the vagina. Vinegar discourages microbial growth and restores acid balance.

+ Frequent use of chlorinated swimming pools and hot tubs can lower the acidity of the vagina.

After menopause, the internal environment of the vagina changes from slightly acidic to alkaline. If you are taking estrogen or antibiotics, or overindulging in sugar and processed foods, this change may be more pronounced. Coupled with the fact that the outer vaginal lips are now smaller and provide less protection for the vagina, urethra, and bladder, infections can begin more easily and spread quickly.

Acidophilus

There are several natural solutions to maintaining and restoring vaginal pH balance. Douching with a plain lactobacillus acidophilus yogurt or powdered acidophilus is quite successful. Add a few tablespoons of yogurt or powder to warm douche water, or, if you prefer, insert several teaspoons of yogurt into the vagina with a tampon and then lie down for 5 to 10 minutes. As yogurt is even more effective internally, add it to your diet to create a beneficial environment in the intestine.

Acidophilus is also available in supplemental form and helps to reestablish friendly bacteria in the colon and detoxify harmful substances. Because it is sensitive to heat, store it in a cool, dry place. Take 1 to 2 capsules on an empty stomach in the morning and 1 hour before meals. Many types and brands of acidophilus are on the market, such as Maxidophilus and Megadophilus. You can even get a milk-free variety, such as Kyo-Dophilus. A nondairy yogurt with live acidophilus is available in most health-food stores and some general markets. Milks and other dairy products are now often fortified with acidophilus. If you are on antibiotics, wait until you have finished the series before taking acidophilus orally.

Cranberry Juice

The urinary tract has built-in defenses against bacterial growth. The lining of the bladder has antimicrobial properties that prevent bacteria from adhering to its surface cells. This is the reason cranberry juice can relieve bladder infections—once again, an example of folk remedies gaining scientific authenticity. Recent studies show that substances in cranberry juice reduce the ability of E. coli (a resident bacteria in the body that can get out of control) to adhere to the walls of the bladder and urethra.(8) The juice of the blueberry also possesses the antiadhesive agents that prevent bladder infections.

At the first indication of infection, start drinking pure, unsweetened cranberry or blueberry juice, or juice sweetened with apple or other sweet juices. Stay away from juices with added sugar or high fructose corn syrup. Ten to 16 ounces a day will probably be enough without irritating your stomach. If the juice is too strong, dilute it with water. Some women find it easier to take 3 capsules of concentrated cranberry juice 3 times a day.

Other Remedies

Drinking plenty of water helps dilute the urine and flush bacteria from the bladder. Cleansing the system with natural diuretics such as celery, parsley, and watermelon also helps to relieve discomfort.

When fighting an infection, stay away from foods and drinks that drain the system rather than build it up: caffeine, carbonated beverages, chocolate, alcohol, and sugar should be eliminated, or at least, kept to a minimum. Eating foods and taking supplements that fight infection may help lessen the severity or prevent frequent recurring symptoms. Vitamin C is known to fight infection. It helps create an acidic environment in the bladder and urinary tract, which discourages bacterial growth. The recommended dosage once infection is well underway is 500 mg every two hours or until you notice loose stools (then decrease the dosage until they return to normal). If you have not yet added a multivitamin and mineral supplement to your diet, now would be a good time to rebuild your defenses.

Garlic, long reported to ward off vampires and witches, also fights infection. With the emergence of more and more new strains of bacteria that are resistant to modern drugs, scientists are once again looking at garlic's infection-fighting capabilities. Scientific studies show that garlic helps to prevent and to treat infections of all kinds. Take it whole, raw, baked, or cooked with vegetables. If you prefer, garlic is available in capsule form; take 3 to 4 a day.

One of the more effective botanical antimicrobial agents for the treatment of bacterial infections is goldenseal. Take 1 teaspoon in a cup of hot water for tea or as a tincture, 3 times a day. You also might try dandelion tea or extract, or bearberry (uva ursi).

EXERCISES FOR ENHANCING YOUR SEX LIFE

Exercising the vaginal, stomach, and back muscles will greatly extend your years of sexual pleasure. Keeping the muscles surrounding the internal organs toned and tight will prevent many common complaints, such as backache, fallen organs, involuntary urination, and excessive dryness. The most commonly recommended exercises are the Kegel exercises. Developed more than 40 years ago, they strengthen the pubococcygeus (PC) muscle, the band of muscle that extends from the pubic bone in front to the coccyx (tailbone) in back. Since the PC muscle supports the vaginal tissues as well as the internal pelvic organs, it requires continual strengthening.

Kegel exercises can be started when a woman is in her teens, although better-late-than-never works just fine here too. They can improve sexual satisfaction, make childbirth easier, and are useful for women of any age who suffer from poor bladder control and leaking urine.

If you are unsure where the PC muscles are, the next time you go to the bathroom, try and stop the flow of your urine. The muscles you contract are the PC muscles. If you try it without urinating, you will be able to exert even more pressure. You don't have to strain to gain benefit, however, so take it easy and breathe naturally when doing the exercises described below. Kegel exercises can be done anytime, anywhere, and there are variations if you tend to get bored doing only one kind of exercise.

Kegel Exercises

1. Contract the PC muscle tightly and hold for 3 seconds, relax for 3 seconds, and repeat. Gradually build to 10 seconds.

2. Contract and release the PC muscle as rapidly as you can, starting with 10 repetitions and working up to 100.

3. A lying-down position works both the PC muscle and the internal organs. Lie on your back, with your knees bent and your feet on the floor. Raise your pelvis until you feel the stretch, and then begin squeezing.

Kegel exercises are the most popular exercises for strengthening and toning the vaginal muscles. However, other muscles in and around the reproductive organs also require strengthening and toning. All of the muscles in front of, behind, and surrounding the female organs work best at protecting the lower body if they are tight and firm.

As with any other muscle, disuse of the vaginal muscle results in diminished tone and decreased flexibility, and eventually atrophies. Many sex therapists recommend regular and frequent intercourse to ensure adequate lubrication, muscle tone, and continued sexual health. Ralph W. Gause, a doctor and sex therapist, observes that the decrease in estrogen and the lack of sexual activity work together: "The estrogen level may fall but if the vagina is sexually active, it remains fully functional."[9]

The enjoyment of sex has more to do with attitude and continued sexual practice than with any of the age-related changes. If you have had a rewarding love life before menopause, you have every reason to believe it will continue. Should temporary symptoms arise, they can, for the most part, be treated with natural methods. A combination of a sound knowledge of the aging process, acceptance of yourself, and an understanding attitude toward your partner will enable you to learn new, creative ways of finding sexual pleasure.

MAINTAINING A HEALTHY BODY FOR A HEALTHY SEX LIFE

A satisfying sex life depends on a healthy body. Sexual function and desire are closely linked to hormone production and the condition of the endocrine glands. To function optimally, all the hormone-producing glands—including the thyroid, pituitary, adrenals, and sex glands—require nutritional support.

Low Thyroid Function

Hypothyroidism may be a cause of low sexual desire. A low meta-bolic rate caused by a sluggish thyroid not only produces fatigue, lethargy, and weight gain, but may be responsible for decreased sexual interest. Conversely, an overactive thyroid (hyperthyroid), which speeds up the body's basal metabolism, can result in ram-pant sexuality. People who take thyroid hormones often report an unusually strong interest in sex. A number of nutrients, such as iodine, copper, zinc, and the amino acid tyrosine, are important in activating the thyroid gland in individuals with thyroid activity.[10]

Certain foods may inhibit glandular secretion and thus sexual interest: turnips, kale, cabbage, and soybeans contain an antithy-roid substance and should be avoided by individuals with decreased thyroid activity. Fasting, although sometimes a healthful practice, may inhibit thyroid function. When the body does not get enough calories, it slows down to conserve energy. Regular fasting may induce a slowed metabolic state and inhibit sexual urges. If you want to increase or maintain your sexual activity, eat regularly.

Exhausted Adrenals

The adrenal glands are critical to sexual development and drive. If you suffer from adrenal exhaustion, which can be caused by con-tinued external stress (death, divorce, moving, family problems), internal stress (overuse of sugar, fat, coffee, or alcohol), or both, you may not feel very romantic. Finding ways of handling stress is vital for a more enjoyable sex life.

Keeping your adrenal glands healthy is important all through life because they assume a starring role at menopause: the primary producers of estrogen. Many symptoms we attribute to meno-pause—fatigue, lethargy, dizziness, headaches, forgetfulness, food cravings, allergies, and blood-sugar disorders—may actually be more related to reduced adrenal function.

If you suspect your adrenals are exhausted, you can revitalize them by providing a respite from both external and internal stress. Start with those things over which you have better control: your food selections. Avoid or reduce (sometimes denying yourself com-pletely can be a far greater stress than minimizing) foods that aggravate and overstimulate the system: concentrated sugars, fried foods, alcohol, caffeine, tobacco, processed foods, and salt. Emphasize fresh, whole, raw fruits and vegetables (foods that are easy to digest), whole grains, and low-fat chicken and fish. Supplementing with a multiple vitamin and mineral tablet will help replace nutrients that have been in short supply and enable your adrenals to rebuild and repair. Exercise also helps to relieve stress and stimulate healthy adrenal function.

Medications

Sexual desire and performance can be adversely affected by many things: certain drugs (tranquilizers, muscle relaxants, antidepressants, amphetamines, diuretics, antihypertensives, and hormones, to name a few), alcohol, marijuana, cigarettes, coffee, overwork, tension, frustration, and depression. The general effects on the body include stress on the adrenal glands and depletion of a wide variety of nutrients.

Vitamin E

Vitamin E is concentrated in the pituitary gland and is essential for the production of sex hormones and adrenal hormones. It is also required for normal brain functioning and muscular reflexes, which are involved in sexual arousal. Acting as an antioxidant, it protects body organs and glands from destruction by oxygen. Vitamin E directly and indirectly touches every cell of the body, protecting them from aging. It is difficult to obtain even the minimum RDA of vitamin E exclusively from food because processing and refining destroy so much. Still, it is good to get what you can from food sources: wheat germ, nuts, seeds, eggs, leafy vegetables, and vegetable oils provide the richest supply. Most people can take up to 400 IU of vitamin E daily; however, if you have a rheumatic heart, diabetes, or high blood pressure, consult with your doctor first.

Zinc

Zinc, like vitamin E, is found in high concentrations in the pituitary gland. Its role as a nutrient involved in sexual enjoyment has to do with its close association with blood histamine levels. Studies have shown that women with low histamine levels are often unable to reach orgasm, whereas women with high blood histamine levels achieve orgasm easily. The higher the histamine level in men, the quicker the ejaculation; and the lower the count, the slower the response. Men and women who take antihistamines regularly need to be aware of the possibility of decreased sexual desire, delayed orgasm, and ejaculation difficulties. Zinc deficiency is common in women because they lose significant amounts during menstruation, and diet often reinforces this loss. Refining grains and cereals removes 80 percent of the zinc, rendering these foods useless as viable sources. The recommended dosage for a healthy sex life is 15 to 30 mg per day, usually supplied in a multivitamin and mineral tablet. Good sources are the following: oysters, beef, turkey, crab, sunflower seeds, almonds, and beans. For the precise amount of this nutrient contained in certain foods, consult Appendix C.

Niacin (Vitamin B-3)

Niacin is another nutrient that may be associated with histamine production. Life-extension researchers Durk Pearson and Sandy Shaw report that niacin not only causes the release of histamines, but also stimulates the formation of mucus in response to sexual activity.[11] Take niacin as part of a multivitamin tablet or B-complex unit, making sure the major B vitamins range between 25 mg and 50 mg. Good sources are the following: tuna, liver, turkey, salmon, beef, brown rice, and enriched bread. For the precise amount of this nutrient contained in certain foods, consult Appendix C.

A good diet is the foundation of a good hormone balance. It not only increases your libido, but it often minimizes the problems of menopause—such as hot flashes, insomnia, and vaginal dryness—that put a damper on your sex life. With those hindrances out of the way, you can begin to enjoy the sexual freedom of your later years.

6

DEPRESSION AND MOOD SWINGS

Sometimes I feel like a figment
of my own imagination.
—LILY TOMLIN

Historically, menopause has been associated with irritability, nervousness, emotional instability, and depression. If a woman of 50 cries or is cranky or melancholy, her feelings are blamed on shifting hormones. This is a harmful attitude. First, it makes a woman feel she has no choice but to give in to her chemical "controls." Second, if she is clinically depressed or if other conditions are responsible, she may postpone seeking appropriate professional help. When emotions cannot be explained, all possibilities need to be examined—family situations, fear of the change or of aging, and health status.

INTERNALLY OR EXTERNALLY INDUCED?

Whether depression and mood swings during menopause are psychological or biological in origin is still hotly debated by scientists and clinical practitioners. Opinions are divided into two main schools of thought, each with profoundly different implications for research and clinical treatment. One viewpoint holds that depression and mood swings are associated with or triggered by endocrine changes at midlife. A second and more recent view holds that these experiences are related to social issues encountered by women in their 40s and 50s.

Studies from different countries, encompassing a broad age range and spanning various socioeconomic strata, reveal that, while depression is common among women, there is no indication that menopausal women are more susceptible than other women. An extensive research project involving approximately 2,500 randomly selected premenopausal women, came to these striking conclusions:[1]

1. Depression was not associated with the natural changes of menopause or with the hormonal changes accompanying the event.

2. The only midlife women who reported depression were those who recently experienced a surgical menopause. The rate in this atypical group of women was twice as high as in the pre- to postmenopause group.

3. The most marked increase in depression was related primarily to events and situations likely to occur in midlife but unrelated to menopause itself.

4. The factor associated most strongly with depression was ill health, as measured by the number of physical symptoms reported. An even stronger association was noted with those people who had recently been diagnosed with chronic conditions.

Other studies show that depression is associated significantly with marital status and education. Widowed, divorced, and separated women with fewer than 12 years of education are the most depressed group. Never-married women have low rates of depression, while married women fall in the middle.

In other words, clinical depression and the less-debilitating mood swings are associated with factors *other* than female hormonal fluctuation. These factors include: physical disorders (underactive thyroid, endometriosis, stomach upset, headaches), nutritional deficiencies, poor lifestyle habits, stress, deprivation of light, lack of sleep, and unresolved psychological issues.

It is important to remember that not all women entering menopause become depressed or sing the blues all day. Some women sail through the change happy, rewarded, and secure—cultural conditioning, hormonal imbalances, and all. Sadja Greenwood, assistant clinical professor at the University of California Medical Center at San Francisco, claims that women who value themselves in their work (as homemakers or in a career), and women who have interesting jobs, steady incomes, a sense of purpose, and things to do usually report fewer problems with menopause.[2] Feeling secure and worthwhile contributes to our physical, as well as emotional, health.

PHYSICAL FACTORS
CONTRIBUTING TO DEPRESSION

Our emotions are strongly affected by the inner climate of the body, and the more dramatic the change in that environment, the more likely we are to feel uneasy. Think about how you feel when you are sick with the flu. You are nauseated, tired, and weak. Everything aches—even your teeth and hair seem to hurt. And as you feel physically drained, your attitude toward the world around you changes. You don't want to talk, you are short-tempered, and your outlook is anything but positive and uplifting. Ill health often leads to a negative emotional state that eases once health improves.

Researchers at Harvard Medical School report that there is a difference in blood hormone levels between depressed and non-depressed people. A sharp drop in hormone levels may lead to significant changes in behavior. Certain women experience greater hormonal highs and lows throughout their lives. Women who have suffered from premenstrual syndrome can testify to the reality of the physical and emotional symptoms they experience when their hormones fluctuate. But just as all women don't have PMS, not all women experience a large drop in hormones at menopause. By maintaining a healthy body in the years prior to menopause, a woman is less prone to the biochemical extremes that can alter behavior.

Biochemical and hormonal factors may induce depression in an otherwise healthy individual. The endocrine and nervous systems are closely linked, and when any hormone—sex-related or not—is out of balance, emotions can be affected. For example, during the first several days and even weeks following the birth of a baby, there is an abrupt decline in circulating estrogen, progesterone, and cortisol in the mother. This, coupled with the physiological drain of labor, causes many women to experience a significant emotional low known as postpartum depression. Even women who have had an uneventful pregnancy and an easy delivery may experience it. I did, and my pregnancy was textbook normal. If some wise woman had told me that uncontrollable crying was to be expected, I probably would have experienced less guilt. Just knowing in advance can relieve anxiety.

The fact is, estrogen affects the brain and central nervous system. As estrogen decreases, brain hormone levels, the ones that make us feel good, also fall. When the drop is abrupt, as with a hysterectomy, chances of extreme mood disturbances increase. This rapid drop in hormones happens in about 15 to 20 percent of women who have had hysterectomies.[3]

If you are in this category, you may want to consider estrogen replacement. If you have had your ovaries removed and are still years from normal menopause age, hormone replacement will improve your symptoms. However, perimenopausal women may or may not find it effective. Some women report elevation in mood with estrogen; others cite no positive changes. Hormone replacement therapy can be both a miracle drug and a nightmare; opinions and individual experiences differ tremendously.

OTHER FACTORS
CONTRIBUTING TO DEPRESSION

Most of us struggle at some point in our lives with periods of feeling unhappy or out of focus. This is not the clinical definition of depression. According to Barbara Edelstein, psychiatric resident at the Eastern Pennsylvania Psychiatric Institute of Living and author of *The Woman Doctor's Medical Guide,* "the depressed person is unhappy, discouraged, pessimistic, wiped-out, bored, guilty, disgusted, clumsy, tearful, suicidal, irritable, disinterested, indecisive, unmotivated, sleepless, sexless, helpless, and hopeless."[4] We can probably all claim some experience with these feelings. The difference is that the truly depressed individual experiences most of these feelings most of the time—and usually to a high degree.

Earlier Unresolved Issues

Depression may not manifest itself more at midlife, but if it does we should not dismiss its significance by masking symptoms with hormones and tranquilizers. Traditional psychology teaches that emotional symptoms reflect an underlying conflict the individual is attempting to resolve. If a woman has not come to terms with a particular issue, such as her own identity, her depression could be a continuing problem that has flared up at midlife. Some psychiatrists believe that menopause, like any other major life event, can stimulate the resurgence of unresolved psychosocial conflicts from earlier stages.[5] If this research had been presented to me eight years ago when I started researching menopause, it would have remained theory to me. However, the events of the past two years shook my reality not just of menopause, but of underlying family issues I had never reconciled. Two years ago, when I was 48 years old, my husband was transferred. Though I wasn't overjoyed at the idea of leaving my children, extended family, friends, church, nutritional consulting practice, and social network, I tried to think of it as "God's calling." Anyone might expect that a major move would take major adjustment, so at first I wasn't overly concerned about my daily crying jags and bouts of staring into space for hours. After a year without much improvement despite genuine attempts to "get over it" by trying all the self-help strategies that had worked so well in the past—exercise, fresh air and sun, long baths, vitamins, and prayer—I knew I needed professional help.

At first, I strongly rejected any suggestion that the experiences of my early years were related to my present sadness. It took the skill and sensitivity of a wonderful therapist to show me how the abrupt loss of my life as I knew it had triggered other, earlier memories of losses that I had ignored and suppressed—childhood wounds that were still festering and needed healing. I never would have dreamed that, at almost 50 years old, I needed to grieve a situation I would rather not even remember. Allen Chinen, author of *Once Upon a Midlife: Classic Stories and Mythic Tales to Illuminate the Middle Years*, believes that confronting and dealing with past traumas is a major midlife task for women and men.[6] When depression is real, there is no substitute for counseling. Hormones, tranquilizers, even exercise and the best diet in the world will not work—at least not for long.

Midlife is a monumental transition for some individuals, and it may be a time when we are forced to confront repressed emotional issues. According to William Bridges in his book *Transitions*, "The transitions of life's afternoon are more mysterious than those of its mornings and so we have tended to pass them off as the effects of physical aging."[7] You might consider that early issues were passed over as you cared for your family and made a living. Even if you think you came to terms with deep-seated hurts, you might examine them again and make sure they are not still eating away at your happiness.

The Role of Self-Esteem

Judging from the higher rates of depression in women compared to men, in both the United States and Europe, it seems women in our culture struggle more than men with role perception and self-identity. Gloria Steinem writes in *Revolution from Within: A Book of Self-Esteem* about the pervasiveness of women's poor self-opinion: "Wherever I traveled, I saw women who were smart, courageous, or valuable, who didn't *think* they were smart, courageous, or valuable—and this was true not only for women who were poor or otherwise doubly discriminated against, but for supposedly privileged and powerful women, too."[8] At some time in our lives, we all need to deal with the question of what we are really worth.

Studies reveal that most women see themselves in terms of either their bodies or their various roles. Psychologist Lillian Rubin found that, when asked to describe themselves, most women started with their physical attributes: "I'm short, tall, blond, fat, pretty, not so pretty anymore, average."[9] One should not find these responses surprising in a culture in which youth and beauty are women's most valued attributes; however, they don't say much about who we really are.

Women who are overconcerned with their physical appearance or have defined their role in terms of husband and children seem to have the most difficulty accepting the change of life. Certain female roles increase the incidence of emotional loss. For example, women who are overprotective of their children are more likely than other women to suffer depression after their children leave home.[10] Mothers who have sacrificed their own dreams to live vicariously through their children are more likely to experience the "empty-nest syndrome" when their children move away.

A woman's emotional life prior to menopause will determine, at least in part, how she will react to physiological changes. If she has not defined her identity as a woman in the years prior to menopause, there is strong evidence that menopause may be a difficult emotional transition. If she has emotional unfinished business, it may bubble up and flood her life. How do you know if your feelings are hormonal or psychological? My experience is, keep your mind open to all the facts and information, and then go with your gut feelings.

FOOD AND MOOD

Food—or the lack of it—has a potent effect on mood, thinking, and behavior. Many women are undernourished due to excessive dieting or poor food selection. Government surveys show that women barely take in half the RDAs (recommended daily allowances), a minimum requirement for health.

Proper functioning of the brain, more than any other organ, is dependent on what we eat. In the early 1970s, Richard Wurtman, a neuroendocrinologist from MIT, found that mood is related to concentrations of certain chemicals called neurotransmitters in the brain and that, by eating certain foods or taking specific nutrients, an individual can raise the level of these brain chemicals and thus feel better.[11] The three neurotransmitters that most influence behavior are serotonin, dopamine, and norepinephrine.

Serotonin

Serotonin is the neurotransmitter known to ease anxiety and promote a sense of well-being. Generally speaking, we can raise serotonin levels in the brain by simply eating carbohydrates. Other nutrients that aid this chemical conversion are the amino acid tryptophan and vitamin B-6. Tryptophan is abundant in proteins such as chicken, seeds, and nuts, and is normally available in the body from previous meals. When carbohydrates are consumed, the increase in insulin removes from circulation other amino acids that compete with tryptophan; therefore, tryptophan easily enters the brain to make serotonin.

Serotonin is produced quickly when we eat starchy foods such as breads, pastas, and cereals. That is why, if you are feeling down, as few as one or two crackers or half a bagel may raise your spirits. Sugar in small amounts also works, but remember that blood-sugar imbalances caused by too much sugar can induce depression. As with most recommendations, there are exceptions. Some women—particularly those who are 20 percent or more over their ideal weight or are premenstrual—may need more carbohydrates to trigger serotonin production.[12] The few carbohydrate-sensitive women may not respond at all to these guidelines. They instead feel more than relaxed after a carbohydrate meal—in fact, they may just go to the couch and fall asleep. Finding out how carbohydrates react in your body is an easy and fun experiment.

Several lifestyle conditions may lower serotonin production and bring you down emotionally. These include stress, overwork, and trauma. Balance and moderation are probably most conducive to feeling good.

Factors That Can Lower Serotonin Levels and Your Mood

+ lowered estrogen levels

+ higher than normal progesterone levels

+ congenital hormonal abnormalities

+ low carbohydrate diet

+ excessive carbohydrates

+ weight fluctuations

+ consuming 80 percent or less of daily RDAs

+ alcohol and drug abuse

+ light deprivation

Dopamine and Norepinephrine

Dopamine and norepinephrine are called psychic energizers because they produce chemicals that stimulate your mind. When the brain produces these, people report thinking more quickly and feeling more alert and motivated—that experience that everything just clicks into place. Eating protein is the prescription for energizing the mind. Whenever you eat a protein in isolation (like a piece of chicken or a hard-boiled egg), or in combination with a small amount of a carbohydrate (as in a sandwich), you allow more of the amino acid tyrosine to reach your brain. Tyrosine, with the help of B vitamins, produces dopamine and norepinephrine. All you need is 3 to 4 ounces of protein to stimulate this conversion.

Endorphins

Endorphins are another class of brain chemical that, when produced in adequate amounts, will make you feel content and happy. The endocrine system and nervous system are closely linked; any sudden drop in hormones is likely to create feelings of anxiety. During menopause, if estrogen drops abruptly, there is a concomitant decrease in endorphins in the central nervous system.

The good news is that there are natural methods to elevate endorphin levels. The most accessible one is exercise. An exercise program that included both aerobic and resistance training increased the concentration of several brain chemicals in menopausal women, including endorphins and serotonin.[13]

Exercise is considered by some more effective in relieving depression than the most commonly used tranquilizers. In 1978, John Grerist, of the University of Wisconsin, found running to be as useful as psychotherapy for depression. Even when the study was over, the once-depressed subjects continued to run, finding that when they quit their depression returned.[14] Running may not be the answer for you but walking is a good alternative, and there are any number of other forms of exercise you can do. If you feel down, get out and start your heart pumping for at least 20 minutes, four times a week. It will undoubtedly raise your spirits.

You may try other approaches to boost your endorphins. Have you ever wondered why menopausal women go ballistic over candy bars and truffles? They elevate endorphin levels. But don't think this gives you license to devour an entire box: all it takes to trigger the endorphin surge is one small ounce. Should you decide to trade in your running shoes for bakeware, remember that exercise is 20 times more effective in raising endorphins than chocolate.

Other practices that may help in raising your spirits are laughing, crying, water submersion (hot baths or tubs), relaxation techniques, acupuncture, sex, coffee, and cigarettes. Obviously, some choices are better—healthier—than others.

Maintaining Blood-Sugar Levels

As discussed earlier, maintaining a constant level of glucose in the blood is important to well-being. The brain and nervous system are especially sensitive to disturbances in blood-glucose levels. The central nervous system does not store glucose, and it needs more of it than any other part of the body. The primary component of that system, the brain, is the first to feel the deficiency when the glucose level is low. The brain and nervous system are so hypersensitive to disturbances of body chemistry that a defect in the utilization of sugar can result in an erratic mental state, with a list of symptoms and complaints that reads like the label on a bottle of snake-oil: dizziness, fainting, headaches, fatigue, muscle pains, cold hands and feet, insomnia, irritability, crying spells, nervous breakdown, excessive worry, depression, illogical fears, suicidal thoughts, crawling sensation, loss of sexual drive—and the list goes on.[15]

The brain is more dependent for proper functioning on what we eat than any other organ. Diets high in sugar, coffee, and alcohol can cause a roller-coaster ride of emotions, especially in the middle years. Tolerance to sugar declines with age, so strong reactions may be noticed after eating foods one was once accustomed to enjoying. Maybe you have already noticed that desserts, espressos, or combinations of food and drink set you off both physically and emotionally, or that going all day without eating no longer serves you well. Be careful about eating on the run or forgetting a meal; it may trigger mood swings.

We all experience sporadic blood-sugar fluctuations at various times in our lives. If you are feeling low and can't explain why, examine your eating habits. Do they include drinking a lot of coffee or alcohol, or eating large amounts of sugar and processed foods? All of these can contribute to unnatural highs and lows. To stabilize your blood-sugar level, eliminate these stresses from your diet and eat foods high in protein and complex carbohydrates.

The number of meals you eat a day can affect your mood as well. Six small meals a day are much more conducive to a slow release of insulin from the pancreas, allowing for the subsequent gradual release of glucose, than three large meals.

NUTRIENTS AND EMOTIONS

Psychological disturbances are some of the earliest symptoms of nutritional inadequacies. The normal production and function of neurotransmitters demands a full range of supporting nutrients. For example, vitamin B-6 is needed in both the conversion of the amino acid tryptophan to serotonin and the conversion of the amino acid tyrosine to dopamine.

Even one deficient nutrient can play havoc with our nervous systems. Roger Williams, the biochemist who discovered pantothenic acid, has done extensive original work in the field of vitamin research. He discusses the importance of nutrients in the control of mental problems, and says the most important way to improve the environment of the brain cells in a threatened individual is to supply her or him with the full nutritional requirements.[16] If you have emotional distress, what are the chances that you are missing a vital vitamin or mineral in your diet? Check whether any of the symptoms listed below are familiar to you.

Nutrient Deficiencies and Related Mental Symptoms

+ *Vitamin B-1 (thiamine):* loss of appetite, depression, irritability, memory loss, sensitivity to noise, inability to concentrate, fatigue, reduced attention span

+ *Vitamin B-3 (niacin):* insomnia, nervousness, irritability, confusion, depression, hallucination, loss of memory

+ *Vitamin B-6:* anxiety, depression, irritability, insomnia

+ *Pantothenic acid:* depression, inability to tolerate stress

+ *Vitamin B-12 (cobalamine):* difficulty concentrating and remembering, stuporous depression, severe agitation, hallucinations, manic behavior

+ *Folic acid:* irritability, weakness, apathy, hostility, anemia

+ *Vitamin C:* increased stress and fatigue

+ *Vitamin E:* depression, lethargy

+ *Potassium:* nervousness, irritability, mental disorientation

+ *Magnesium:* paranoid psychosis

+ *Calcium:* anxiety, neurosis, fatigue, insomnia, tension

+ *Zinc:* anemia, poor mental function

+ *Iron:* depression, lethargy, poor concentration, irritability, decreased attention span, personality changes

+ *Essential fatty acids:* anxiety, irritability, insomnia

The chemical makeup of the brain requires an ample and constant supply of essential nutrients. Vitamins, amino acids, fatty acids, and enzymes are all interrelated, each dependent on the others for absorption and utilization; moreover, a shortage of one vital element can render all the others less effective. That is why nutritionists urge people to eat a *variety* of nutrient-dense foods.

HERBAL REMEDIES

A number of herbs have been proven to calm anxiety and reduce tension. It is advantageous to use herbs in conjunction with positive changes in nutrition and lifestyle.

Ginkgo biloba has been widely prescribed in France, Germany, and other European countries to improve blood flow to the brain. Hundreds of studies have substantiated the ability of ginkgo biloba to improve mental health. A recent study indicated it actually improves transmission of nerve signals and is capable of relieving symptoms such as depressive moods, anxiety, tiredness, confusion, poor memory, absent-mindedness.[17] The recommended dose is 40 mg 3 times a day; take it 4 to 6 weeks before expecting results.

Passion flower is another of nature's safe, natural tranquilizers. It relieves anxiety, insomnia, restlessness, muscle tension, and headaches due to nervous tension. Mix 14 to 15 drops of extract in liquid as needed. Some people find it causes drowsiness, so do not drive after taking it. *Do not take during pregnancy.*

Skullcap has been known for centuries for its calming effect on the body. Also called "mad dog weed," it is a traditional remedy for rabies. As an antispasmodic, skullcap has been used to relieve menstrual cramps and muscle pain due to stress. Take 1 capsule up to 3 times a day. If using an extract, mix 3 to 12 drops in liquid and take once a day, or brew a tea mixing 1 tablespoon of the herb with 1 cup of boiling water.

Other helpful herbs to make you feel better are chastetree (vitex), oat straw, Siberian ginseng, dandelion root, garden sage, and chamomile.

Natural Ways to Improve Mood
(Rule out physical illness and psychological issues first)

✦ Maintain even blood-sugar levels.

✦ Practice moderation in sugar, alcohol, drugs, coffee (highly sensitive people may have to eliminate one or all).

✦ Do not overindulge in food.

+ Eat small carbohydrate meals and snacks for relaxation.

+ Eat proteins for mental alertness.

+ Do not try to lose more than 1 to 2 pounds per week if you are dieting.

+ Exercise a minimum of 20 minutes 4 times per week.

+ Expose yourself to the sun or bright, full-spectrum light every day.

+ Take hot baths or lounge in a hot tub for 20 minutes.

+ Learn relaxation techniques.

+ Laugh.

+ Cry.

+ Try acupuncture.

+ Take a multiple vitamin and mineral supplement daily.

+ Use natural herbs.

7

OSTEOPOROSIS

Scientists agree that adequate nutrition
can reduce the impact of osteoporosis
by as much as one half or more.
—JOURNAL OF THE AMERICAN DIETETIC
ASSOCIATION, JUNE 1994

Osteoporosis, a bone-thinning disease that leads to fractures and disability, affects 25 million Americans. Along with heart disease and breast cancer, it is one of the three most serious diseases affecting women. Half of all women between the ages of 45 and 75 show beginning signs of osteoporosis; one in three of these women have full-blown osteoporosis, and, by age 75, the number jumps to 9 in 10 for extreme bone deterioration.[1] Despite these grim statistics, osteoporosis is for the most part preventable. Scientists now agree that adequate nutrition can cut these figures in half and possibly even more.

Osteoporosis literally means porous bones, or bones filled with tiny holes. It is not clinically considered a disease, but rather the progressive and severe loss of bone mass. Because of the loss in density, osteoporotic bones fracture more easily and heal more slowly. While some softening of the bones is normal in both men and women who are of middle age and older, weakness to the degree that one cannot function properly is not normal. In women, the loss of bone begins sooner and proceeds six times more rapidly than in men (primarily because women's bones are smaller).

Our bones are made of living tissue that is continuously recycled. While the inner bone is breaking down, the outer surface is reforming. A delicate balance of the two processes is maintained in response to the demands of the body. If the body needs calcium, bone is broken down; if it doesn't, bone is rebuilt. When more calcium is withdrawn from the bones than is deposited, bones become soft and weak. Reversing this process is the primary step in preventing and treating osteoporosis. There is confusion and conflict about specific recommendations, however, because of the numerous factors that contribute to bone health: genetic predisposition, hormonal output, nutritional status, age, physical activity, and lifestyle habits. It is necessary to examine all the factors involved in this complex problem.

Osteoporosis is expensive. The average cost for two weeks of hospitalization after a hip fracture is roughly $10,000 not including home care and rehabilitation expenses. In the United States alone, more than $1 billion is spent each year for the care and treatment of women with osteoporosis in general.[2]

The severity of the problem cannot be overemphasized. Osteoporosis is painful and crippling. After menopause, a woman's chances of fracturing a bone increase dramatically; even a minor fall or vigorous hug may lead to a break. Bone fractures often result in immobilization, hospitalization, and dependence—and, in extreme cases, even death. Hip fractures are associated with long-term disability and an accelerated death rate. Between 15 and 20 percent of women die within three months of a serious hip fracture; about 30 percent die within six months either of the injury or secondary complications, and those remaining are at risk for recurring fractures or permanent disability.[3]

The physical deformities caused by this condition cannot be concealed: an older woman with advanced osteoporosis loses height, is hunched over, has a protruding abdomen, and often walks with a shuffling, unsteady gait. As the bones of the spine lose density, the vertebrae collapse, forcing the rib cage to tilt downward toward the hip. A curvature in the upper spine creates a second curve in the lower spine pushing the internal organs outward. The stomach protrudes so prominently that the woman may look pregnant.

Because of the compression in the spinal column, up to eight inches in height can be lost. The resulting "dowager's hump" is one of the classic stereotypes of the aging woman—and unfortunately it is not a myth.

As the compressed organs shift positions and put pressure on other organs and systems, internal functions may be impaired. Constipation becomes a problem, and breathing may become labored. Aches and pains throughout the body, particularly in the lower back, may arise from pressure on the nerves emanating from the collapsed vertebrae. Life becomes a series of problems.

A woman's appearance and self-esteem may change drastically when osteoporosis reaches an advanced stage. Along with being uncomfortable and, to varying degrees, incapacitated, she tends to feel awkward, unattractive, and old. Clothes don't fit properly, and a fashionable look is next to impossible. Realizing that the body can never fully return to its premenopausal shape, many women with osteoporosis experience stress, anxiety, feelings of helplessness, and dread of the future. Psychologically, the loss of self-esteem and the emotional adjustments weigh heavier than the physical inconveniences.

DIAGNOSING OSTEOPOROSIS

Osteoporosis is difficult to detect early because it sneaks up gradually. Often, the first sign is a broken bone. The standard x-ray technology used to identify other bone fractures is not sensitive enough to detect osteoporosis until the disease has taken up to 40 percent of bone mass. More sophisticated tests are available, however, to evaluate potential risks at an earlier stage. There are several bone mineral density (BMD) tests on the market that you might consider if you are a candidate for osteoporosis or if you want to establish a benchmark for evaluating your rate of bone loss as you develop your plan of preventive action. Blood and urine tests can help to determine rates of bone loss and formation and to monitor the effectiveness of treatment.

The following early physical warning signs might alert you to a potential problem:

+ chronic low back pain

+ loss of height

+ nocturnal leg cramps

+ joint pain

+ transparent skin

+ rheumatoid arthritis

+ restless behavior (foot jiggling, hair twisting)

+ insomnia

+ tooth loss

+ periodontal (gum) disease

A combination of these symptoms may be a reason for taking the next step for further diagnosis.

WHO IS AT RISK?

Are you at risk for osteoporosis? If you answer yes to two or more of the following questions, continue reading and see what you can do to prevent further bone loss.

Are You at Risk?

+ Has any member of your family had bone disease?

+ Are you short, thin, and small-boned?

+ Are you fair-skinned or freckled?

+ Were your ovaries removed before age 45?

+ Did you have an early, natural menopause?

+ Have you ever given birth?

+ Are you a diabetic or hypoglycemic?

+ Are you lactose intolerant or do you avoid dairy products?

+ Do you have an underactive thyroid gland?

✦ Do you have celiac disease, kidney disease, or liver disease?

✦ Are you sedentary?

✦ Do you drink more than two cups of caffeinated beverages per day?

✦ Do you have more than two alcoholic drinks per day?

✦ Do you smoke cigarettes?

✦ Have you been involved in prolonged dieting or fasting?

✦ Is your diet high in salt?

✦ Do you take in adequate calcium, magnesium, and vitamin D?

There are enough indicators that we can guess, with a fair degree of accuracy, who will or will not develop osteoporosis.

Genetic Predisposition

Let's start with genetic inheritance. If a woman's mother, aunt, or sister incurred fractures because of weak bones, the woman probably will too. I do not agree, however, that we have no control in such a situation. A family tendency toward osteoporosis does not mean that a woman must suffer fractures. Her relatives may have unknowingly aggravated their conditions. Were their diets poorly balanced? Did they take medications or have preexisting medical conditions? Were they active or sedentary? As I discuss in this chapter, lifestyle is key to both preparing for and coping with osteoporosis.

Body Size

Body size is a valuable clue in evaluating risk. Small-boned, thin women—women who wear petite sizes—have a dramatically greater risk than larger women, simply because they have less bone to lose. It is the same reason why men are less susceptible to breakage. Bones respond to a higher weight load by forming new bone tissue to meet the demand: the heavier you are, the greater the stress on your body, the more bone is formed. Research suggests that those who weigh less than 140 pounds have increased chances of developing osteoporosis. However, this should not be interpreted as a case for being overweight, which carries far greater health risks than this benefit. Exercise can provide the same weight-bearing advantages as a larger body.

The inadequate nutrition that is often the cause of thinness, and the lack of estrogen resulting from inadequate body fat, predisposes young women to osteoporosis. Studies show that women and girls suffering from anorexia, bulimia, and other eating disorders already have decreased bone mass.[4] Amenorrhea, the lack of menstrual periods due to inadequate body fat, causes estrogen production to stop and increases the risk of bone loss. Young athletes often fall into both these situations. The numbers are staggering: eating disorders, and their consequences, involve 50 percent of all competitive runners; 44 percent of ballet dancers; 35 percent of noncompetitive runners; and 12 percent of swimmers and cyclists.[5] These shocking statistics help explain why researchers refer to osteoporosis as a childhood disease with a midlife outcome.

Skin Pigmentation

The fairer your complexion, the greater your risk of bone loss. Studies of different ethnic groups have shown that women with northern European ancestry, such as English, Dutch, or German, are at greater risk for osteoporosis and women with African-American ancestry are at the least. Women of Hispanic and Jewish origin appear to fall somewhere in between.

Premature Graying of the Hair

A puzzling risk factor for osteoporosis is premature gray hair (meaning that half the hair has turned color by the age of 40). Scientists at the Maine Center for Osteoporosis Research found that subjects with no identifiable risk factors but with graying hair were 4.4 times as likely to have *osteopenia* (lower than normal bone mass) than those who maintained their natural color.[6] The researchers suspect that the genes controlling early color change are the same as, or close to, those that control bone density. Other possible conditions associated with premature graying are thyroid disease and premature menopause, both contributors to bone loss.

Premature Menopause

Women who undergo premature menopause (before age 45) have a more rapid decline in bone tissue than women who experience menopause naturally. The relationship between osteoporosis and estrogen became clearer during those years when hysterectomies routinely included removal of the ovaries. Surgeons now try to avoid removing the ovaries of premenopausal women to help prevent premature bone deterioration.

Medical Conditions

Medical conditions may make us vulnerable to bone deterioration. Diabetes, kidney or liver abnormalities, celiac disease, Chron's disease, hypothyroidism, and stomach surgery are some of the common medical conditions that, for different reasons, impede absorption and utilization of calcium and other important nutrients necessary for the building of bone.

Bone recycling is a complex process involving interactions of organs, hormones, and minerals. Any defect or disease that affects the nutrient transport system, endocrine system, liver, or kidney functioning, or any illness that requires extended bed rest, causes calcium loss and consequent bone loss.

Medications

Several medications interfere with calcium absorption. Some can easily be avoided; others cannot. Ask your doctor how your prescription drugs affect calcium balance. If you must take any of the following drugs, ask about the advisability of calcium supplementation.

✦ **Corticosteroids** (cortisone, hydrocortisone, prednisone, dexamethasone): Used extensively, these can cause severe bone porosity leading to osteoporosis. They not only create a negative calcium imbalance, but suppress the formation of new bone.

✦ **Anticonvulsants** (phenytoin, phenobarbital, primidone, phensuximide): These stimulate the production of enzymes that break down vitamin D, leading to deficiencies of both vitamin D and calcium, and, in turn, severe bone loss.

✦ **Antacids containing aluminum**   These cause an increase in calcium excretion. Aluminum-containing antacids do not cause osteoporosis per se, but they can be a contributor if taken on a regular basis. Check the label when buying antacids—or anything, for that matter. A few antacids that do not contain aluminum are Alka-Seltzer, Bisodol, Eno, Titralac, and Tums.

✦ **Diuretics**   Women often take diuretics to reduce blood pressure and body fluid. Some are thought to have an adverse effect on bone mass. Long-term usage may cause the blood-calcium level to rise and the excretion of calcium to fall. Morris Notelovitz, director of the Center for Climacteric Studies in Gainesville, Florida, writes that Furosenide increases urinary calcium excretion, while Thiazide reduces the amount of calcium lost in urine and thus is more appropriate for osteoporosis-prone women.[7]

Lifestyle Factors

The speed with which our bones break down depends on the way we treat our bodies: what we regularly put into them and how much we use them. Virtually everything we do is, in one way or another, related to bone health.

Protein

Many studies of societies around the world have proven a correlation between diet and advanced bone disease. For instance, a vegetarian diet helps prevent osteoporosis. Especially after the age of 50, heavy meat eaters lose almost twice as much calcium as do vegetarians. A number of medical investigators have found that consumption of high levels of protein, in excess of 120 grams per day, may stimulate bone resorption (breakdown) and encourage long-term bone loss.[8] One possible explanation is that meat is rich in phosphorus, which accelerates calcium depletion from bone. Protein intake beyond what our body needs also creates acidity in the stomach, a condition that leaches calcium from the skeleton.

Protein, of course, is essential to health, but excess protein leads to chemical imbalances and adverse symptoms. If you have been a heavy meat eater in the past, I strongly urge you to de-emphasize meat in your diet and to add more rice, beans, vegetables, and pasta dishes. You might try thinking of meat more as a condiment than a main course.

Plant-based Alternatives

A soy-based diet appears to be advantageous for preserving bone. Soy protein does not cause calcium excretion like animal protein. In one study, subjects who ate protein from soy sources excreted about 50 mg less urinary calcium than those eating protein from animal sources.[9] Soy foods like tofu and tempeh are rich sources of calcium and phytoestrogens. Recent work suggests that the isoflavones in soybeans also have a direct benefit on bone health, possibly by inhibiting bone resorption.[10] Women from cultures that consume large amounts of soy-based foods do not experience many of our common menopausal symptoms.

As discussed in earlier chapters, many herbs encourage hormone production. Black cohosh, hops, sage, sweetbriar, alfalfa, buckwheat, horsetail, roses, and Shepherd's purse promote estrogen production; chaste tree (vitex), sarsparilla, wild yam, and yarrow promote progesterone production. These natural sources of both estrogen and progesterone can be incorporated into your regimen for building bone. Plant phytosterols are safer than synthetic hormones. They encourage your own body to produce small amounts of hormones—but no more than what you need. Unlike estrogen replacement therapy (ERT) or hormone replacement therapy (HRT), excess dosages are not a worry. In fact, researchers have found that the phytoestrogens, such as are found in tofu, have a protective effect on breast tissue.

Fats

Both the amount and the kind of fat you eat affect calcium absorption. If fat consumption is too high or too low, calcium absorption is depressed. This has been a major criticism of weight-loss diets that call for nonfat milk and other fat-free products. Calcium requires the presence of *some* fat for its absorption, so for the sake of your bones, don't eliminate all fat from your diet, even when you want to lose weight.

A certain amount of fat is needed every day for functions that cannot be performed by any other nutrient. Essential fatty acids are necessary for the metabolization of calcium, and must be obtained from food. The preferred forms of fat are those found in whole natural foods, such as raw seeds and nuts, vegetable oils, and fish. Butterfat in fermented products such as yogurt and acidophilus milk encourages calcium absorption. Even people who are sensitive to milk can usually tolerate these because they are partially predigested.

The fats to avoid—those that alter digestibility and utilization of nutrients—are saturated fats such as those found in meat, dairy products, shortening, processed foods, and certain vegetable oils, such as coconut and palm oil. And keeping fat-calorie intake to no more than 25 percent of the total calorie intake is generally healthy.

Sugar

Those of us with a penchant for sweets run a greater risk of developing osteoporosis. A high sugar intake encourages acidity, which causes calcium to be excreted from the bones. Imagine the effects on your body of being both a voracious meat eater and a sugar fanatic!

Salt

Most people know that excess sodium can raise blood pressure and increase the risk of hypertension and heart disease. Few people realize that too much salt brings another risk: the loss of large amounts of calcium from the bone. The more salt you eat, the more calcium you excrete. It is recommended that daily sodium intake not exceed 1 teaspoon or 2,000 mg. Watch out for hidden offenders: condiments and dressings, processed and canned foods, cheese, hot dogs, cured meats, and pizza.

Caffeine

Coffee, cigarettes, and alcohol all react in the body to produce bone porosity. Young women who drink the equivalent of 2 cups of coffee a day are putting themselves at risk for osteoporosis in later life, according to a study of 980 postmenopausal women.[11] Caffeine acts as a diuretic, speeding up the loss of calcium and magnesium from the body. This study also showed that it is possible to balance the harmful effects of caffeine by adding 8 ounces of milk a day, or the equivalent of 300 mg calcium to the diet.

Alcohol

Heavy alcohol intake has been linked to inadequate absorption of calcium, so most nutritionists counsel high-risk individuals against drinking. This is probably because alcohol has diuretic effects, but it also damages the liver, interfering with vitamin D metabolization. A British study rather surprisingly has suggested that alcohol might increase bone mass, since it causes the conversion of androgens to estrogen.[12] I think the rule of moderation applies to alcohol as it does with other substances that can harm us when we overindulge.

Cigarettes

Female smokers lose bone faster than female nonsmokers. Smokers generally experience menopause several years earlier than nonsmokers, and the premature drop in estrogen may be responsible for diminished absorption of calcium into the bones. Cigarette smoking may also interfere with the body's metabolization of estrogen, although the mechanism by which this happens is unclear. Smoking frequently accompanies consuming caffeine or alcohol—a combination that may be worse than the sum of the individual parts.

THE EXERCISE CONNECTION

There is no controversy concerning the benefits of exercise in building and maintaining strong bones. Like muscle, bone grows stronger with use. Bone density depends directly on how much the bone is stressed: as stress on the bone increases, the amount of calcium deposited in the bones increases. Bones of athletes and physically active individuals are considerably denser than the bones of those who do not exercise.

You don't have to be a marathon runner to get results. Muscle-strengthening exercises, like the ones pictured at the end of the book, help reverse the decline in muscle mass and muscle strength that comes with aging, and may increase bone density. Research at the Center for Climacteric Studies in Florida showed that postmenopausal women on hormone therapy experienced an 8-percent increase in bone mass when they performed muscle-strengthening exercises.[13] A comparison group of women who were on estrogen replacement therapy (ERT) but didn't exercise neither gained nor lost bone mass. Even in a group of 90-year-old women, high-intensity resistance training was found to increase muscle strength and reduce the risk of osteoporotic-related falls.[14]

It doesn't require an unreasonable time commitment to realize results. In a research project at Nassau County Medical Center in New York, postmenopausal women who exercised for one hour three times a week not only stopped losing calcium but actually added some to their bones.[15] The amount of exercise does relate to the amount of increased bone mass. Women who exercise four times a week will have denser bones than those who exercise two times a week.

Osteoporosis is a multidimensional problem, and the many factors that contribute to bone loss must be evaluated as part of a preventive or recovery program. In a recent study of older women it was found that exercise alone was not as effective as exercise plus calcium. In the women who exercised and took calcium, bone loss nearly stopped. Among the women who took estrogen while exercising, bone density increased about 3 percent a year, but this may not be an option for all women.[16]

It is never too late to improve your body. If you are not physically active, start a program as soon as possible, if for no other reason than to protect your bones from deteriorating. The best exercises for bone strengthening are those that put a load on your bones: jogging, aerobic dance, skipping rope, brisk walking, stair climbing, dancing, and strength training. To benefit fully, exercise for 20 to 30 minutes at a pace fast enough to accelerate your pulse moderately. If you suffer from arthritis or other joint problems, consult with your physician first and use your own judgment as to the appropriate type of exercise for you.

Frequently, women concentrate on aerobic exercises or exercises for the lower body and ignore the upper body. This is why so many women have relatively weak arms and shoulders. For a thorough workout, put all your bones and muscles through their full range of movement. Walk or dance for the lower extremities, then add arm and shoulder exercises or work out with weights. Strength training can even be practiced sitting down or in a wheelchair.

Remember that domestic activities, such as gardening and housework, also help to maintain physical fitness. The more you move your body, the healthier you will be—and the fewer physical complaints you will suffer.

Prevention is the best—and for some the *only*—way to avoid the skeletal fractures, severe discomfort, and permanent disfiguration of osteoporosis. Once detected, osteoporosis can be controlled and reversed only to a limited extent, so the safest course is to begin preventive measures now; exercise will add mass to your bones and possibly years to your life.

THE ESTROGEN CONNECTION

The important role of estrogen in bone health has been recognized for decades. Estrogen improves calcium absorption and reduces the amount excreted in the urine. More recent studies show that ERT also protects the heart by decreasing the dangerous LDL (low density lipoprotein) cholesterol levels while elevating the good HDL (high density lipoprotein) cholesterol.

So, why the controversy if it takes only one small tablet a day to be free from the fear of broken bones and protected from heart disease?

For starters, not all women are candidates for ERT. Women with cancers of the uterus and estrogen-related cancers, endometriosis, uterine fibroid tumors, high blood pressure, liver and gallbladder diseases, diabetes, migraines, or a tendency toward blood clotting, for example. Other women find hormonal therapy intolerable because of such side effects as anxiety, mood swings, fluid retention, weight gain, abdominal bloating, withdrawal bleeding, nausea, and headaches.

A growing number of women just don't feel comfortable with the idea of taking hormones and drugs to control a natural life process. Even if there is a chance that the therapy is protective against bone loss and heart disease, the unknowns concerning the long-term effects, such as the possible risk of uterine and breast cancer, disturb many women enough for them to hold off. Some women prefer not to expose themselves to other potential life-threatening diseases, especially if they are not at risk for osteoporosis and heart disease. There are natural, less invasive practices that offer similar protection.

THE PROGESTERONE CONNECTION

Synthetic progesterones, correctly known as progestins, are now added to estrogen to counter some of the problems with using estrogen alone. Researchers report that the combination of both hormones, or hormone replacement therapy, reduces the risk of uterine cancer.[17] For menopausal women who still have a uterus, it is the current treatment. While it appears that HRT relieves some of the concerns, there are still unknowns. Whether this combination has a similar protective effect on breast cancer risk has not yet been confirmed. And adding progestin to estrogen negates the cardio-protective effects of estrogen.

Side effects—depression, moodiness, breast tenderness and enlargement, increased appetite, and headaches—turn many women off to HRT. Sometimes experimenting with smaller doses and different types of hormones will help discomfort; sometimes it won't.

The decision to take hormones should not be made casually. I am not unequivocally against the use of hormones at menopause, but I am against the indiscriminate dispensing of any drug without careful consideration and a very good reason. If you are at high risk for osteoporosis or heart disease, if your body is forced into premature menopause, or if you are suffering unbearable hot flashes or a dry vagina that makes sex intolerable, HRT is an option to seriously consider—but check out the natural methods before you decide. And remember, just because you decide to take hormones, you are not necessarily committed to them for life. You can taper off your use of hormones as you learn better lifestyle and nutritional habits.

Natural Hormones

Most of the hormonal treatments on the market are synthetic, but a growing number of doctors believe that if natural products were used, medical risks and side effects would be considerably lessened. Research using hormones from natural sources is sparse, but some preliminary studies show that natural hormones have the same benefits as synthetics but fewer side effects. A significant finding showed that the adverse effects of the synthetic progestins on blood-fats and cholesterol levels were eliminated with natural progesterone.[18]

John Lee is one of the pioneers testing natural progesterone. He explains in his book *Natural Progesterone: The Multiple Roles of a Remarkable Hormone* that progestin is not progesterone at all. The pharmaceutical companies alter the molecular structure so it no longer fits into the biochemical machinery of the body. Natural progesterone, taken from the wild yam, is nearly identical to what a woman produces and thus is easily converted into the identical molecule within the body.[19]

Dr. Lee and others are also suggesting that progesterone—not estrogen—is the key to building bone. While estrogen can stop bone from deteriorating further, it cannot reverse the process and *build* bone unless progesterone is also present. Since 1982, Lee has treated postmenopausal women with a natural progesterone cream plus a dietary program that includes vitamin and mineral supplements and moderate exercise. He found true reversal of osteoporosis even in patients who did not use estrogen supplements.[20] Lee says that supplementing with the wild yam shows none of the side effects of the synthetic progestins and imposes no increased risk of breast cancer, uterine cancer, or cardiovascular disease.

Natural progesterone cream is available in some pharmacies and health food stores. It is generally applied to the skin in small amounts, in the early morning and before bedtime. For more information on ERT, HRT, and natural hormone products, see the Resources section.

ERT and HRT continue to raise controversy in female health. The best a woman can do is stay informed, continue to question, and find out what best suits her needs. Whether or not hormones are indicated for you, an appropriate diet and lifestyle are still important for preventing osteoporosis, and they have no negative side effects.

THE CALCIUM CONNECTION

The process that ends in osteoporosis begins 30 to 40 years before the first fracture. The early years are when you build bone health; the longer you wait, the harder it is to catch up. Prevention is the best—and the only certain way to maintain bone health. And the story begins with calcium. Getting the calcium in the bones and keeping it there is the trick, and it is not as easy as drinking a glass of milk before bedtime.

To say that calcium is important to the body is an understatement. Because calcium is instrumental in brain function, blood clotting, and muscle contraction, the body is equipped with an elaborate system of hormonal checks and balances to ensure that an adequate amount is circulating in the bloodstream at all times. When blood-calcium levels fall, special hormones and glands respond immediately by withdrawing whatever is needed from the faithful storehouse, the bones.

An adequate amount of calcium in the blood is essential for ensuring that continual withdrawal does not leave the body, decades later, with weakened bones. Many researchers

Calcium Sources

FOOD	PORTION	CALCIUM CONTENT
Nonfat or low-fat (2%) milk	1 cup	300 mg
Sardines (with bones)	¼ lb.	300
Frozen yogurt	1 cup	200
Yogurt	1 cup	290
Cheddar cheese	1 oz.	205
Ice cream	½ cup	190
American cheese	1 oz.	175
Spinach, cooked	1 cup	150
Tofu	4 oz.	145
Broccoli, cooked	1 cup	130
Almonds	¼ cup	80

have concluded that the RDAs are too low for calcium, not just for menopausal women but for children and young adults as well.[21] According to the National Institutes of Health, the daily calcium intake for adult women should now follow these guidelines:

Women aged 25 to 50	1,000 mg
Pregnant women	1,200 mg
Postmenopausal women who are on HRT	1,000 mg
Postmenopausal women who are not on HRT	1,500 mg
Women over 65, whether or not they are on HRT	1,500 mg

In preventing and treating osteoporosis, we need to consider three issues: (1) Are we getting enough calcium in our diets? (2) If we are, what may be preventing us from absorbing the calcium for building bone strength? (3) Is supplementation necessary?

Taking calcium into the body in the form of food should be a top priority, but there are factors that mitigate against it. Some women simply do not drink milk or eat cheese; dairy products don't agree with some women any longer. It is possible they can no longer digest milk; this is true for the majority of African Americans and Asians, who are lactose intolerant. If you would like to get more of your calcium from dairy products, you can try lactaid milk or add enzyme drops to the milk. I have found rice and soy milks to be good with cereal and in cooking, and both are now fortified with calcium.

Dairy products, however, may not be the answer to the calcium question and to bone health. The hip fracture rate is the highest in Western countries, where dairy is consumed in large quantities.[22] Incorporating more of the other food sources of calcium may be better, but consider some of the top contenders: sardines (with the bones), boiled turnip greens, and almonds. Be honest—how many times a week would you really eat these foods? My favorite calcium-rich food is broccoli, but I would have a difficult time forcing down 12 cups to get my daily recommended requirement. Check the following list and add up your approximate daily calcium score.

Consuming calcium-rich foods is only the beginning of the story that takes calcium through the digestive system, into the blood, and to the bones. Since calcium is poorly absorbed by the body, you may need even greater amounts to compensate for the inefficiency. While absorption of any nutrient varies with the individual, at best only 20 to 40 percent of the calcium you ingest is usable and even that percentage decreases with age. Consider some of the complex aspects of calcium absorption:

+ Your genetic makeup determines whether or not you are an efficient absorber.

+ Disease and illness decrease the amount retained.

+ Estrogen enhances calcium absorption, which helps explain the rapid loss of bone after menopause.

+ Calcium absorption declines with increasing age in both men and women, but the decline begins earlier for women.

+ Exercise increases absorption; inactivity decreases it.

+ Medications, drugs, cigarettes, caffeine, and certain foods impede absorption, increase excretion of nutrients, and decrease utilization.

+ Stress depletes your immediate supply as well as your storehouse of calcium.

+ Lack of other specific nutrients will deter absorption, especially vitamins D, C, K, and the minerals magnesium, phosphorous, and boron.

Supplementation, then, is absolutely necessary and is proven to be effective in reducing bone loss in postmenopausal women.[23] Choosing which supplement to buy can be frustrating. Calcium carbonate is clearly the most popular and widely available source, largely because it contains the most *elemental*, or actual, calcium; however, it is not the best choice for the mature woman. Calcium citrate is the preferred form, since it is better tolerated by individuals with low stomach acid, a condition common among older adults.[24]

The safety of certain calcium supplements has also been questioned. For several years health educators have warned the public about dolomite and bone meal because they contain the toxic metals lead and cadmium. Recently, significant amounts of lead and aluminum have been found in one of the more popular sources of calcium, the calcium carbonate labeled "oyster shell" or "natural source."[25] Calcium citrate does not contain these metals.

Absorption of calcium is enhanced when calcium intake is spread out over the day. Dole out your portions and take them with each meal. If you forget to take calcium during the day, be sure to remember at night, when bone loss is greatest.

Many women ask about the superiority of name brands over generic products. In the case of calcium, the National Osteoporosis Foundation *does* recommend that you stick to brand-name supplements. There is a way to test for quality and dissolution time. Drop one tablet into a small container of vinegar. If it takes more than 30 minutes to dissolve, shop elsewhere.

NUTRIENTS THAT BUILD STRONG BONES

Our information about the interrelationships among nutrients constantly expands. Bone health involves not just calcium but an array of cofactors.

Vitamin D

Vitamin D is vital to calcium absorption. Without it the small intestine cannot absorb calcium adequately no matter how much there is available. A lack of vitamin D has been found in 30 percent of postmenopausal women with bone deterioration.[26] Vitamin D and calcium can inhibit hip fractures even after 80 years of age. This is the finding of a research project directed by a team of French scientists who set out to see if they could prevent bone fractures in a group of over 3,000 ambulatory women living in nursing homes. For 18 months, half of these women were given daily supplements of 1.2 grams of calcium and 800 IU of vitamin D; the other half received inactive tablets. At the end of the study, the women receiving the vitamins had a 40 percent lower rate of hip fractures and 32 percent lower incidence of wrist, arm, and pelvic fractures. The scientists noted few side effects and concluded that calcium plus vitamin D was a safe and effective way to prevent fractures.[27]

Sunlight is the most effortless way to promote the manufacture of natural vitamin D in the body. Just 30 minutes a day of direct exposure is all that is necessary for the skin to convert a type of cholesterol into vitamin D. If this is not possible for you because you live where there is little sun, or you usually stay indoors or cover yourself outdoors, or you are exposed to sunlight primarily through a window or screen, then supplementation as part of a multivitamin and mineral program may be worthwhile. Good dietary sources of vitamin D include: salmon, tuna, shrimp, fortified milk, and egg yolks. For the precise amount of this nutrient contained in certain foods, consult Appendix C.

Vitamin C

Vitamin C is necessary for the manufacture of collagen, a fibrous protein that is found in connective tissue and cartilage and is essential for proper bone formation. Since the need for collagen regeneration increases with age, vitamin C is needed in greater amounts as one gets older. With age, the stomach tends to produce less acid. Vitamin C also facilitates the absorption of calcium by creating the weak acidity level necessary for proper digestion. Good sources include: kiwi fruit, raw green peppers, orange juice, broccoli, grapefruit juice, watermelon, and grapes. For the precise amount of this nutrient contained in certain foods, consult Appendix C.

Vitamin K

Low blood levels of vitamin K—the form that is found in green leafy plants (kale, collard greens, lettuce, and parsley)—were found in patients with fractures due to bone loss. The more severe the fracture, the lower the level of circulating vitamin K.[28] The RDA for vitamin K is 70 to 150 mcg. Good sources include: broccoli, lettuce, cabbage, spinach, and asparagus. For the precise amount of this nutrient contained in certain foods, consult Appendix C.

Magnesium

The mineral magnesium is instrumental in converting vitamin D to its usable form and in keeping calcium soluble in the bloodstream. A magnesium deficiency disturbs the calcification of bone, impairs bone growth, and reduces calcium. Tests have shown that diets deficient in magnesium can lead to skeletal abnormalities, including osteoporosis.

Calcium, vitamin D, and phosphorus all increase magnesium requirements, thus emphasizing the importance of nutrient inter-relationships. Evidence suggests that the balance between calcium and magnesium is especially important. If the calcium level is raised, magnesium intake must be raised as well. The optimum calcium/magnesium ratio is two to one; thus, if you are taking 1,000 mg of calcium, you need 500 mg of magnesium. Calcium and magnesium are available in the correct proportion in single tablets. Good sources of magnesium include: peanuts, Bran Buds, lentils, tofu, wild rice, bean sprouts, and chicken. For the precise amount of this nutrient contained in certain foods, consult Appendix C.

Daily Nutritional Support for the Prevention and Treatment of Osteoporosis

NUTRIENT	AMOUNT
calcium	1,000 mg before menopause; 1,500–2,000 mg after
vitamin D	400–800 IU
magnesium	500 mg before menopause; 750–1,000 mg after
vitamin C	60–1,000 mg
vitamin K	150–500 mcg
boron	3 mg

Phosphorus

Phosphorus is necessary to metabolize calcium, but deficiency of the mineral is uncommon. Anybody who eats a typical modern-day diet of red meat, white bread, processed cheeses, soft drinks, and packaged pastries gets more than his or her quota of phosphorus.

The ratio of calcium to phosphorus affects the amount of calcium absorbed by the bones. Ideally, the balance should be two to one in favor of calcium. With the abundance of phosphorus found in today's foods, the balance has tipped four to one in favor of phosphorus. Not only is this change not conducive to calcium retention, it accelerates bone demineralization by stimulating the parathyroid glands, which secrete a bone-dissolving hormone called parathyroid hormone.

To reestablish the correct mineral ratio, reduce your intake of high-phosphorus foods drastically. Concentrate on eliminating processed foods, which often offer little nutrition anyway. These include almost all processed or canned meats (hot dogs, luncheon meats, bacon, ham, sausage), processed cheeses, instant soups, puddings, packaged pastries, soft drinks, breads, and cereals. Check the labels of packaged goods for ingredients such as sodium phosphate, potassium phosphate, phosphoric acid, pyrophosphate, or polyphosphate; if you find them, put the products back on the shelf.

Boron

Boron, a mineral needed in very small amounts in our bodies, has gained attention as another protective factor against osteoporosis. Supplementing the diet of postmenopausal women with 3 mg of boron a day reduced urinary calcium excretion by 44 percent and dramatically increased the levels of the most usable form of estrogen. In its active form, boron also appears to activate vitamin D conversion. Fruits and vegetables are the main dietary sources of boron and, typically, American diets are deficient. Only 10 percent meet the minimum requirement of these foods.[29]

Other nutrients that may be instrumental in building bone include zinc, copper, manganese, and silicone.

8

BLEEDING, CRAMPS, PMS, BREAST DISEASE, INSOMNIA, ARTHRITIS— AND THE GOOD LIFE

From month to month, from birth to the
giving of life to the change of life,
women face a unique challenge to
keep their body chemistry in balance.
—RICHARD KUNIN
MEGA-NUTRITION FOR WOMEN

The majority of women do not experience a major disruption in their lives due to menopause, although many are temporarily bothered by a number of physical concerns. Getting appropriate treatment during midlife years appears to be more challenging than at any other time in a woman's life. Depending on a physician's attitude and clinical experience with women going through the change, a woman's symptoms may be overtreated, undertreated, or misdiagnosed. If the doctor views menopause as a hormonal deficiency disease, unnecessary medications may be prescribed. On the other hand, some physicians regard all complaints as hormonal and may overlook something more serious.

In defense of the medical community, when real symptoms surface at menopause, diagnosing whether the problem is due to hormonal changes, some undetected physical abnormality, or the natural aging process can be challenging. When questions arise over a symptom, inform yourself about natural signs of menopause, consult medical professionals to rule out any functional cause, and then make an educated decision about the best course of action for you.

HEAVY BLEEDING (MENORRHAGIA)

Erratic periods with heavy bleeding is a common perimenopausal symptom. If an egg is not released for a month or more and progesterone is not produced, estrogen continues to build up the uterine lining. Finally, the sheer bulk of the blood-rich tissue causes an especially heavy flow, which may also be accompanied by large clots. Long, profuse periods can be uncomfortable and a bit frightening. Some women report periods of up to 10 days with flow so continuous that the combination of a tampon and a super-absorbent pad cannot contain it. The amount of blood lost over a week can be draining and may cause extreme fatigue.

Heavy or continuous bleeding is occasionally a symptom of something more serious, such as uterine fibroids, polyps, and in rare cases, uterine or cervical cancer. Should your heavy bleeding last for more than a few months, check with your physician.

Many doctors prescribe progestins to compensate for the body's reduced production of natural progesterone. By preventing the buildup of the endometrial lining, progestins create a more regular monthly period and relieve excess bleeding. They do not, however, alleviate bleeding in all women, and some women find the side effects of depression, fatigue, bloating, and breast tenderness too unpleasant to continue. Not all physicians are aware that there is a natural progesterone cream on the market that carries all of the benefits of the synthetic variety, but without the side effects. For more specific information about natural hormones, see the Resources section.

Unexpected bleeding can be scary, but if it is temporary, it is usually a sign of hormonal changes. Nutritionally, there are several important remedies that will help you feel better and build up your body during periods of excessive blood loss.

Iron

Blood loss is well known as a major cause of iron-deficiency anemia. It is not as well known that chronic iron deficiency can itself cause menorrhagia, or severe bleeding. Iron deficiency may be the most prevalent nutritional deficiency in the United States, and women, throughout their lives, are at risk because of their increased need.

Iron comes in two dietary forms. Heme iron, the most efficiently absorbed, is found in red meats, egg yolks, and fish. Nonheme iron, the plant variety, comes from grains, beans, and dried fruits. It must be ionized by stomach acid and then transported by a complex mechanism before it can be used by the body; thus absorption is more tricky. Lack of stomach acid makes this more of a challenge for menopausal women, and blocking agents such as fiber, phosphates, and preservatives prevent absorption. If you shy away from meat, you can enhance absorption of your vegetarian sources by taking in a vitamin C source at the same time. Good sources of iron include: liver, clams, oysters, beef, shrimp, poultry, prune juice, almonds, raisins, spinach, and split peas. For the precise amount of this nutrient contained in certain foods, consult Appendix C.

Supplemental iron may be required to replenish low iron stores because it is difficult for women to eat enough iron-rich foods. A daily dose of 100 mg elemental iron has been used therapeutically to treat excessive bleeding.[1] Liver extracts provide an excellent source of heme iron; take two 500 mg capsules with meals. Several nonheme iron supplements on the market are also very good; those bound to ascorbate, succinate, fumerate, glycinate, or aspartate are better absorbed and tolerated. Take these forms on an empty stomach unless they causes you discomfort, in which case take them with meals.

Vitamin C and Bioflavenoids

Vitamin C not only aids in iron absorption, it, along with bioflavenoids, has been tested as a treatment for heavy menstrual bleeding. Both nutrients effectively decrease menstrual flow by strengthening capillary walls. Increase your fruit and vegetable intake, especially emphasizing blueberries, grapes, cherries, and blackberries. It will take a considerable effort to eat enough to reach suggested dosages, so supplement with vitamin C (1,000–4,000 mg) and bioflavenoids (500–2,000 mg) per day as needed.

Vitamin A

Vitamin A is important for the support and restoration of the skin and mucous membranes including the vaginal and urinary tissues. Deficiencies often result in alteration in both skin and mucous membranes that resemble precancerous conditions. This finding has promoted more research into vitamin A as a possible anti-cancer agent or cancer preventive. Studies show that women who bleed excessively have significantly lower levels of vitamin A than women with more moderate periods, and that treatment with vitamin A normalizes blood flow.

The best sources of vitamin A are a wide variety of fruits and vegetables that contain beta carotene, which is converted in the body to its active form. While vitamin A from animal sources can produce toxicity in large amounts, beta carotene is completely safe even in high doses. Recommended dosage is between 25,000 IU and 50,000 IU per day. Good sources include: liver, carrots, sweet potatoes, pumpkin, spinach, cantaloupe, papaya, and watermelon. For the precise amount of this nutrient contained in certain foods, consult Appendix C.

B Vitamins

As far back as the early forties, medical literature recorded that B vitamins were instrumental in regulating estrogen levels in the liver.[2] When B vitamins are insufficient, estrogen levels escalate. Furthermore, excess estrogen creates B-vitamin deficiency, and a vicious cycle ensues. Since heavy menstrual flow can be caused by excess buildup of estrogen in the body, it is imperative to keep adequate amounts of B vitamins circulating in the system. Dietary sources of many B vitamins include whole grain products, desiccated liver, brewer's yeast, wheat germ, beans, and peas. For women with heavy periods, the amounts needed to create a therapeutic benefit cannot be met by food alone. Supplement with a multivitamin and mineral tablet or a B-complex tablet containing at least 50 mg of B-1, B-2, and B-6.

Essential Fatty Acids

Essential fatty acids, fats that our bodies require but cannot manufacture, can normalize heavy periods. Sprinkle 1 to 2 tablespoons of the following on salads or vegetables or take 2 to 8 capsules per day: borage oil, black currant seed oil, flaxseed oil, evening primrose oil. Store these sources of EFA in the refrigerator, and do cook with them.

Herbs

Several herbs can be useful in relieving profuse menstrual flow. Dandelion leaves contain an absorbable source of iron and are used to prevent iron-deficiency anemia. It is also a natural diuretic and digestive aid and enhances liver and gallbladder function. Take 1 capsule up to 3 times a day or mix 10 to 30 drops of liquid extract in juice or water.

Vitex (chaste tree) and wild yam root both can stimulate progesterone precursors to stabilize hormones and remedy excessive bleeding. Take in capsules (1–3 divided throughout the day) or in tincture form (20–25 drops several times a day) for several months.

MENSTRUAL CRAMPS

Monthly cramping during perimenopause intensifies in some women and subsides in others. The culprit is a substance called *prostaglandin*. When menstrual cramps are accompanied by nausea, vomiting, diarrhea, fatigue, tension, and headaches, the sufferer is probably producing greater than normal amounts of this hormonelike chemical. The reason for this overproduction has not yet been determined; my own bias leads me to suspect that nutrition is involved.

Diet

Several researchers have found a strong correlation between hormone imbalances and vitamin and mineral deficiencies, and most menstrual problems seem to be caused by hormonal imbalances. When the nutritional deficiency is corrected by diet or supplements, hormone levels often return to normal.[3] This suggests that a lack of proper nutrients can result in a wide array of symptoms.

A diet of primarily complex carbohydrates and calcium-rich leafy green vegetables, especially the week before the period, seems to help many women. Holding off on sugar, caffeine, and red meats generally works well too. If this is not enough to relieve your cramps, supplement with a multivitamin and mineral complex that includes a B-complex (10–30 mg), vitamin C (100–1,000 mg), vitamin E (400 IU), calcium (1,000–1,500 mg), magnesium (500 mg), zinc (30–60 mg).

Exercise

If you are bothered by cramps, remember that vigorous exercise four or five times a week will help prevent them. Exercise forces deep breathing, which brings more oxygen to the blood, relaxing the uterus and raising endorphin levels to relieve pain naturally. Yoga, stretching, and long hot baths relax the body, allowing tension and pain to recede.

Cramp Bark

Cramp bark, as its name implies, is one of the best herbal remedies for menstrual cramps. It acts to reduce muscular tension and spasms and has also been used for threatened miscarriages. Some of its properties are aspirinlike and help to reduce general pain. Make a tea of cramp bark using 2 teaspoons of the dried bark or herb in 1 quart of boiling water, and simmer for 15 minutes. Drink up to 3 cups a day. If you prefer powdered capsules, take $\frac{1}{2}$ gram to 1 gram three times a day. Caution: do not take cramp bark if you are on blood-thinning drugs because it also works as a blood thinner.

Other herbs that ease menstrual cramps include vitex, ginger, and garden sage. Make a tea or down a capsule for convenience.

PREMENSTRUAL SYNDROME

For years I refused to admit, even to myself, that my minor recurring irritability and outbursts were in any way related to my menstrual cycle. Eventually, I discovered, first through research and then through experience, that my PMS symptoms were brought on or exacerbated by the foods I chose. For me, the amounts of sugar and coffee I was consuming were more reflective of my symptoms than the time of month: I was being controlled by my eating habits, not my hormones. Today, whenever I revert to my old coffee and cookie habit, I recreate my PMS symptoms. Some may argue that I did not have classic PMS, and perhaps this is true. But many other women are also on the fringe of PMS, so to speak, and can be helped through dietary and supplemental assistance.

PMS has generated widespread interest among medical researchers and practitioners around the world. Clinics have cropped up, books are increasingly available, and new products are being formulated. Doctors are experimenting with a variety of theories about the causes of PMS, from the hormonal, biochemical, and neuroendocrinologic to the psychological and psychosocial. Possible causes being explored include an excessive amount of estrogen, a deficiency of progesterone, an imbalance of prolactin, excessive amounts of prostaglandins, hormone allergies, decreased endorphins, hypoglycemia, various vitamin and mineral deficiencies, abnormal metabolization of essential fatty acids, stress, and psychological factors. There is not enough scientific data to establish one theory above all others. What clouds the issue is that no single treatment works for all women: some women respond to progesterone therapy, some to dietary changes, and others to placebos.

This suggests that PMS is a condition involving a host of interacting factors. The treatment you require will depend on your circumstances. (The treatment you get will probably also depend on your doctor's prejudices.) Before undergoing hormonal therapy you may want to try the safest and least invasive methods: diet, nutritional supplements, and exercise. Diet and exercise alone will not work for every woman, but they may be the only remedy for some and will at least help minimize symptoms in most.

The connection between nutrient deficiencies and hormonal imbalances works something like this: without adequate nourishment our endocrine glands cannot manufacture hormones in normal quantities. Nutritional deficiencies also lower the threshold for stress, increasing the hormonal imbalance.

How Can You Be Sure You Have PMS?

Even this point arouses controversy. The classic definition is that if you have one or more regular, recurring physical and psychological symptoms one or two weeks prior to menstruation that improve after the onset, you are a likely candidate. Katharina Dalton, a physician who has written extensively on the subject, emphasizes "It is the absence of symptoms and the change of mood after menstruation back to being a happy, energetic, vivacious woman once more, which clinches the diagnosis."[4]

There are currently no definitive medical, hormonal, or psychological tests available for PMS. The diagnosis remains a subjective one, most likely made by the woman herself. Symptoms include irritability, mood swings, depression, hostility, confusion, coordination difficulties, fatigue, food binges, headaches, fainting, bloating, weight gain, constipation, acne, joint pain, and breast tenderness, to name a few. In fact, more than 150 symptoms have been associated with premenstrual syndrome.

Most experts agree that the best method for determining whether or not you have PMS is to keep a daily record of your symptoms for three months. You may use a calendar you have, design your own, or use one of the professional charts put out by various authors and groups. If you are using a home calendar, mark down the date your symptoms occur and when you menstruate. I suggest you also chart your food intake; this information will be a significant help in establishing necessary dietary changes.

Diet

Certain foods provoke and aggravate premenstrual symptoms; they should be eliminated a week or two before menstruation and minimized the rest of the month.

Red-Light Foods for PMS Sufferers

+ *Sugar, alcohol, caffeine, tea, and cigarettes:* PMS women are often hypoglycemic, so maintaining a consistent blood-sugar level is important.

+ *Red meats:* These are high in fat (which decreases the liver's efficiency in metabolizing hormones) and in phosphates (which use the body's calcium).

+ *Salt and high-sodium foods:* These increase water retention and cause breast tenderness.

+ *Dairy products:* These interfere with magnesium absorption and are high in sodium and fat.

+ *Cold foods and drinks:* These can contribute to cramping by reducing abdominal circulation.

In addition to reducing your intake of foods that aggravate PMS, increase your consumption of foods that encourage relief of symptoms. Beneficial foods include complex carbohydrates, such as whole grains, vegetables, beans, rice, and fruits. Since fluid retention is widespread among women with menstrual problems, drinking at least two quarts of water each day will help. Natural diuretics such as watermelon, strawberries, artichokes, asparagus, watercress, and parsley will also help.

Essential Fatty Acids

Essential fatty acids are important for women during all stages of life and can specifically reduce cramps and other monthly symptoms. Evening primrose oil (EPO), which is richly supplied with an essential fatty acid, has been tested both in the United States and England. British studies have found that EPO relieved PMS in two thirds of women who were not helped by any other means; another 20 percent were greatly improved.[5] EPO has also been found useful in treating women with heavy and prolonged menstrual bleeding and women suffering from fibrocystic breast disease.

EPO is by far the richest source of gammalinoleic acid (GLA), one of the building blocks from which the body creates a

Daily Nutritional Supplements and Their Potential Effects on PMS

NUTRIENT	EFFECT
B complex (10–30 mg)	Regulates estrogen activity
vitamin B-6 (50–300 mg)	Reduces water retention; calms nervous tension; preserves higher levels of magnesium
magnesium (500–2,000 mg)	Normalizes glucose metabolization; produces calming effect
calcium (1,000–2,000 mg)	Reduces pelvic pain, insomnia, bloating, nervousness
vitamin E (200–600 IU)	Reduces breast pain and tenderness; normalize production of sex hormones; acts as a mild prostaglandin inhibitor
vitamin C (500–1,000 mg)	Reduces allergic response; relieves pain
lecithin (1 teaspoon)	Helps prevent excessive fatty deposits in liver; deactivates estrogen
zinc (30–50 mg)	Improves glucose tolerance; helps regulate prostaglandins

prostaglandin called PGE1. A deficiency of PGE1 allows the hormone prolactin to become excessive in the body. Prolactin is another hormone found in greater than normal amounts in the PMS woman.

To be effective, EPO must be taken daily. The six to eight capsules, along with 50–200 mg of vitamin B-6 (pyridoxine), should be divided into two or three doses during the day. Vitamin E (100–600 IU) plus the other nutrients involved in the biochemical conversion process are generally helpful and can be found in a multivitamin and mineral tablet. Start slowly, with smaller doses, and increase as necessary. Remember, too, how slowly the body environment changes. Two to three months is not an unreasonable length of time to wait before noticing results.

EPO is expensive, so I was pleased to read that Richard Kunin has found that the EFAs in fish oils are just as effective in treating PMS. As little as 10 grams or 2 teaspoons of salmon oil a day can be effective.[6] Other good sources of the necessary EFAs include flax oil, wheat germ oil, borage oil, and omega-3 fish oils. Diabetics should not take supplemental fish oils, but can eat more cold water fish, such as salmon, tuna, trout, herring, and sardines.

Other Supplements

Many supplements designed specifically for PMS can be found in retail and health food stores. If you are taking multiple vitamins, check to see that you are getting at least the minimum therapeutic doses of the following nutrients.

Dong quai is an all-purpose herb for PMS, painful periods, cramps, hot flashes, and other symptoms related to hormonal fluctuations. Rich in vitamins and minerals, it is also taken to treat insomnia, anemia, and high blood pressure. Take 1 to 3 capsules a day, or drink 1 to 2 teaspoons in 8 ounces of hot water.

FIBROCYSTIC BREAST DISEASE

Fibrocystic breast disease, also called cystic mastitis, is the most common noncancerous breast condition among women. It is not a disease per se, but a growth of fibrous tissues that most frequently appears when a woman is in her late 30s or 40s and disappears with menopause. Fibrocystic breasts are uncomfortable, but the condition is not serious. Some 20 percent of the female population may, at some time in their lives, develop breast tenderness, swelling, discomfort, or noticeable lumps.

Breast cysts are influenced by the menstrual cycle and hormonal fluctuations, enlarging and becoming more painful just prior to the onset of the period. An imbalance in the estrogen/progesterone ratio seems to be responsible for both the cysts and the enlargement, but whether the important factor is the overproduction of estrogen or the underproduction of progesterone is not yet agreed upon by scientists.

Certain situations that result in a shifting hormonal balance may bring on FBD; it has been found in teenagers who have not achieved regular menstrual periods, women who have children late in life, women who have gained weight, women on estrogen treatment, and women under stress. Pregnancy and breastfeeding tend to improve the condition, as does menopause—unless, of course, estrogen hormone is taken.

Breast lumps are common and are usually a problem only because they are difficult to distinguish from cancerous lumps. A lump that fluctuates with your period usually indicates a harmless cyst. If you are past menopause, check the lump at the same time each month. (If you have FBD, you will continue to have cystic changes in your breasts even though your periods have stopped.) If your lump does not move, have a gynecologist examine your breast.

There is no sure way to reduce breast lumps, but dietary intervention has been found to help. John Minton, professor of clinical oncology at the Ohio State University College of Medicine, found a connection between chemicals called *methylxanthines* and FBD. When a group of women with FBD abstained from coffee, tea, chocolate, soft drinks, and various drugs, all of which contain methylxanthines, 65 percent became free of breast lumps in one to six months.[7]

Caffeine

Since Minton's study, other researchers and clinicians have had similar success. Penny Budoff conducted a test on herself and some of her patients who had premenstrual breast tenderness. Abstaining from coffee, they all felt they had better months—less pain, less irritability, and milder cramps.[8]

Vitamin E

Supplemental vitamin E, at levels of 400–800 IU per day, has been found effective in the treatment of breast tenderness. In a study in which vitamin E was combined with reduced consumption of the xanthine compounds, improvement was found in 85 percent.[9] This should be good news for drinkers of coffee and black tea who are suffering from breast tenderness: you can reduce your intake of xanthine compounds by reducing—or giving up entirely—your consumption of these liquids. Other dietary remedies for FBD that help some women are cutting down on fat, salt, and cigarettes.

B-complex Vitamins

The B-complex vitamins regulate estrogen activity by promoting healthy liver function. Early studies show that when women supplement their diets with the B vitamins, they find relief from symptoms related to excess estrogen, including heavy menstrual flow, PMS, and fibrocystic breasts.[10] B vitamins can easily be taken as part of a multivitamin and mineral tablet.

INSOMNIA

Sleep patterns are commonly interrupted during the transition years. Hot flashes and night sweats may wake us from a sound rest; frequent trips to the bathroom disturb us and keep us from going back to sleep. Many women report that bad dreams and unsettled feelings prevent them from getting adequate rest even when they do sleep. One night, maybe even a few nights, like this may not be noticeable, but repeated episodes leave us drained, unable to think and act clearly, and often lead to depression and mood swings.

Blood-Sugar Levels

Evaluating one's lifestyle, activities, and food intake is the first step to combating sleeplessness. The kinds, amounts, and timing of foods and drinks you consume may prevent you from falling asleep or wake you during the night. Eating a large, heavy, fatty meal after 9:00 P.M. is a sure ticket to catching the late night movie. It is hardly news that the caffeine in coffee, chocolate, sodas, and tea can keep one alert until dawn, but it may not be known that alcohol does not stimulate restful sleep. While you may fall asleep quickly after several glasses of wine, its diuretic action will awake you several times during the night.

Erratic blood-sugar levels interrupt sleep. The brain is highly dependent on glucose (sugar) as an energy source, so a drop in blood sugar may trigger a wake-up call. Some people can handle moderate amounts of sugar with relative ease; others do not. With age and overworked adrenal glands, our ability to tolerate extremes may be impaired. Many factors other than overindulgence in sugar can contribute to blood-sugar fluctuations, and remember, the higher the high, the lower the low.

Maintaining an even blood-sugar level throughout the day and night is necessary if you want a good night's sleep. The diet recommended is no different from what is healthful for most situations: high in complex carbohydrates, high in fiber-rich foods, low in fat, and moderate in protein. A few extremely sensitive individuals must reduce starches in favor of more protein, but most individuals only have to adjust amounts and timing of meals. It is important to eat small meals or snacks often (about every 4 hours) and to avoid overindulging in concentrated sugars (even fruit juices for the highly sensitive), caffeine, alcohol, and refined, processed foods. Exercise will help stabilize hormonal levels, and a good multivitamin and mineral supplement will ensure that nutritional errors will not aggravate the condition. A chromium supplement of 200 mcg improves glucose tolerance, helping to regulate blood-sugar levels.[11]

Serotonin

Serotonin, a brain neurotransmitter, regulates mood, pain, eating habits, and sleep. The synthesis of serotonin within the brain is dependent on the availability of tryptophan (an amino acid), the ingestion of a starchy food, and the cofactors vitamin B-6 and magnesium. Short-term insomnia might be helped by eating a nighttime snack of foods rich in tryptophan, such as milk, yogurt, tuna, turkey, almonds, bananas, or peanut butter. Accompany this snack with a piece of bread or a few crackers, and crawl under the covers.

Vitamin B-6 levels are often under par in women, especially those who are on the Pill or who take ERT. All the B vitamins are involved in maintaining a healthy nervous system, so when even one is lacking, symptoms of anxiety, nervous tension, and insomnia result. While the recommended daily allowance (RDA) is 2 mg per day, many health professionals recommend doses between 50 mg and 200 mg. Do not exceed 300 mg a day of vitamin B-6, as studies have found that, in some people, higher levels may result in damage to nerve tissues. Good sources of B-6 include: bananas, avocado, hamburger, cheese, fish, potatoes, and spinach. For the precise amount of this nutrient contained in certain foods, consult Appendix C.

Another B vitamin, B-3 (niacin), may be useful for women who fall asleep but later wake up. Like the other B vitamins, niacin functions in more than 50 body processes, but it also has a specialized effect for calming the nerves. Niacin can be produced in the body from the amino acid tryptophan. Again, the interrelationship of the vitamins, amino acids, and brain chemicals points out the importance of optimum diet to good health. Studies indicated that one type of niacin, niacinamide, has an action similar to that of a low-dose tranquilizer: supplemental doses of between 50 and 100 mg may help you to get to sleep and stay asleep.

The other form of niacin, nicotinic acid, is regarded as one of the substances of choice for lowering blood cholesterol levels. Those who take therapeutic doses over 100 mg experience a burning sensation in the face and neck and other side effects including nausea, headaches, cramps, and altered heart rate. Larger doses of nicotinic acid (over 2,000 mg) may result in liver toxicity. At these levels, it must be prescribed and monitored by a physician. Good sources of these vitamins include: chicken, salmon, beef, peanut butter, and peas. For the precise amount of this nutrient contained in certain foods, consult Appendix C.

The full complex of B vitamins is vital for maximum benefit to the nervous system. Because they are water soluble, they readily pass through the system and constantly need replenishment. Take the full complex in a multivitamin tablet; for specific purposes, take the single B vitamin. Many people find that taking B vitamins too close to bedtime is too energizing so try to work them in at breakfast or lunch.

Magnesium, the second cofactor needed for the transformation of tryptophan to serotonin, also functions in muscle relaxation, contraction of nerve transmission, and conversion of food to usable energy. Menopausal women need

Causes of Blood-Sugar Fluctuations

INCREASES BLOOD SUGAR	DECREASES BLOOD SUGAR
overeating	skipping meals
concentrated sugars	endurance exercise
alcohol	alcohol
stress	stress
infection, surgery	large doses of aspirin
estrogen	anabolic steroids
cortisone	barbiturates
lithium	beta blockers
thiazide	blood-thinning drugs
nicotine	
caffeine	

400 to 750 mg a day to ensure these jobs get done. Magnesium is best taken together with calcium in a 2:1 ratio of calcium to magnesium, and is available in supplements in the correct ratio. Adding more magnesium-rich foods to your diet is still a good idea. Good sources of magnesium include: peanuts, split peas, tofu,

cashews, fortified breakfast cereal, spinach, beef, and milk. For the precise amount of this nutrient contained in certain foods, consult Appendix C.

Medications

Medications frequently contribute to sleeping problems. Check your prescriptions and over-the-counter labels. A few common drugs that interfere with restful nights are appetite suppressants, decongestants, high-blood-pressure medications, and pain relievers and cold remedies that contain caffeine. Strangely, even drugs that help you sleep and calm you can eventually reach a point in your body where they not only are ineffective but trigger the opposite reaction.

Herbs

Many plants have sedative actions in the body. Consult an herbalist for ones that might work best for you.

✦ **Passion flower**   Hailed as one of nature's best tranquilizers, passion flower relieves anxiety, muscle tension, restlessness, and headaches. Since tryptophan was taken off the market because of one contaminated batch, passion flower has become its replacement for promoting sleep. You can steep the dried herb for tea or mix 15 to 50 drops of extract in liquid as needed. Do not take before driving or operating heavy machinery.

✦ **Valerian**   Tagged as the "valium of the nineteenth century," valerian is recognized worldwide for its relaxing effect on the body. Recent studies have substantiated valerian's ability to improve quality sleep and relieve insomnia.[12] Unlike many prescription drugs, valerian is not addictive and has no side effects, except for a bad taste. Forget the tea—take it in capsule form, 2 grams two hours before bedtime and another 2 grams at bedtime. Don't take valerian continuously for more than two weeks.

Exercise

Regular physical exercise improves sleeping habits as well as general well-being. It is best not to work out too close to bedtime, as it may be a long time before you feel relaxed enough to even get into bed. Relaxation techniques before bed and a hot bath may also be soothing.

JOINT PAIN AND ARTHRITIS

Aching hands, creaking knees, sore ankles, and a tired back are common complaints of menopausal women. Whether it's age or hormones, body aches and pains seem to show up in women who have not experienced them before or intensify in women who have.

Inflammation of the joints has many causes, including injury and complications from another disease. It may occur sometimes as a side effect of medications, such as contraceptives, anticonvulsants, and major tranquilizers. There appears to be a strong relationship between arthritis and diet: eating certain foods and eliminating others often results in relief from pain.

The two most common types of arthritis are rheumatoid arthritis (RA) and osteoarthritis (OA). RA attacks at any age and is characterized by inflammation, not only in the joints but also in the connective tissue throughout the body. The body replaces the damaged tissue with scar tissue, creating stiffness, swelling, fatigue, fever, weight loss, anemia, and often crippling pain. The onset of RA may be associated with physical or emotional stress; however, poor nutrition or bacterial infection may be factors as well.

OA is the most common form of arthritis and appears in later years. It is a degenerative disease related to the wear and tear of aging and involves deterioration of the cartilage at the ends of the bones. The joints most likely to be affected are those of the feet, toes, and fingers, and the joints of the weight-bearing bones, such as the knees, hips, ankles, and backbone. The onset of OA can be subtle, with morning joint stiffness often the first indication. As the disease progresses, there is pain when the joint is active that is worsened by prolonged motion and relieved by rest. Unlike RA, disablement is usually minor and swelling minimal.

Dietary Recommendations

Inadequate dietary intake of certain vitamins and minerals is associated with RA, although it is unclear whether poor nutrition is a cause or an effect of the disease. Some people, though, are clearly helped by a diet that minimizes saturated fat, sugar, meat, and alcohol, and emphasizes more complex carbohydrates from vegetables, beans, and whole grains. Fresh, unprocessed, raw fruits and vegetables are of paramount importance because they are rich sources of pain-relieving nutrients, including vitamin C, the carotenes, and bioflavenoids. Even if complete relief from pain is not realized, this diet will make you feel better in other ways and improve the quality of your health.

✦ **Lose excess weight**   Probably the best dietary advice for anyone with arthritis is to maintain a normal body weight for your age. Excess weight increases stress on the weight-bearing joints, increasing pain. This recommendation alone can greatly ease discomfort and stiffness.

✦ **Include sulfur-rich foods**   A sulfur-bearing amino acid found in garlic, onion, eggs, beans, brussels sprouts, and cabbage seems to alleviate pain and swelling of joints. Interestingly, a large study in the mid-1930s found the sulfur content of the fingernails of arthritis sufferers to be lower than that of nonsufferers.[13] This research has never been pursued, though others testify to its validity.

✦ **Some fats are good**   We usually associate fat with ill-health; however, some fats actually prevent and control the inflammation (and subsequently, pain) of arthritis. Prostaglandins are important contributors to the inflammatory process, and specific fatty acids can modulate their production. Diets rich in omega-3 fatty acids (fish oils), taken in supplemental form, have been shown to reduce inflammation in both OA and RA. When 10 capsules of the fatty acid EPA (eichosapentaenoic acid) were given to patients with RA, noticeable improvement was found in joint tenderness and morning stiffness after 12 weeks, while the control group worsened.[14]

The recommended dosage of EPA is 2,000 to 3,000 mg daily. Diabetics should not take supplemental fish oils, but can eat more cold-water fish such as salmon, tuna, trout, herring, and sardines. Another way to maintain essential fats is to incorporate more plant sources in your diet, such as flaxseed, pumpkin seeds, walnuts, and green leafy vegetables. Fortified flax is particularly good;

mix 1 tablespoon with water or juice, or add it to salads, yogurt, and cereals.

Some evidence has shown that gamma-linolenic acid (GLA), an essential fat from the omega-6 family found in evening primrose oil, may also be useful in some types of arthritis. It is thought that a lack of GLA may lead to a dysfunctional level of prostaglandins. The recommended dosage is 1 to 2 g per day of GLA or evening primrose oil. These oils are found naturally in raw seeds and nuts like flaxseed, pumpkin seeds, sesame seeds, sunflower seeds, and walnuts.

✦ **"No" to the nightshade family** Sometimes it's not what you do eat but what you don't eat that can improve your health. Elimination of an entire food group is a simple dietary change that has worked for some arthritis sufferers. Some research suggests that susceptible people might develop arthritis, as well as a variety of other complaints, from long-term, low-level consumption of the alkaloid-containing "nightshade" plants: tomatoes, potatoes, eggplant, peppers, and tobacco.[15] Presumably, alkaloids inhibit normal collagen repair in the joints or promote the inflammatory degeneration of the joints. It may be worth your experimenting if you suffer with OA or RA.

Food Allergies and Arthritis

It has long been suspected that RA may result from or be exacerbated by a food allergy or sensitivity. Completely eliminating or minimizing certain common foods, therefore, may also reduce symptoms. Food allergies have been tested and found to aggravate many of the aches and pains associated with arthritis. In a well-controlled experiment, a hypoallergenic diet produced marked improvements in 75 percent of the subjects.[16]

An *allergy* is an inappropriate response by the body's immune system to a substance that is not normally harmful. The manifestations of such an overreaction are varied: diarrhea, gastric upset, bloating, fatigue, headache, hives, acne, itching, ear infections, rapid heartbeat, shortness of breath, muscle pain or weakness, hypoglycemia, anxiety, mental confusion, inability to concentrate, and vision changes. What strikes me as I read over this list is the number of symptoms that are also thought to be menopausal.

Wouldn't it be ironic if all we had were allergies, which flared up at this particular time?

Any food is a potential allergen, but the most common are wheat, milk, corn, soy, yeast, chocolate, tea, coffee, beef, citrus fruits, shellfish, eggs, and potatoes. To determine if you are sensitive to any of these, first consider how often you eat them. It is more than coincidental that the foods you crave may be the ones to which you are also be sensitive. The body's reaction to food allergens is similar to addiction.

It is possible to test for allergies without expensive treatments. The most effective method is to fast without food or juices for three to five days and then reintroduce one food at a time into your diet. Symptoms are usually obvious, leaving little doubt as to the offending food or foods. If going without food is not an option, try plan B. Eliminate a suspected food, such as dairy or wheat products, for two weeks or more, then reintroduce it into your diet and watch for symptoms. It is best to test one food at a time, as you may be sensitive to more than one.

There is another way of detecting a possible food intolerance. First, take your pulse several different times for one full minute to determine your resting pulse rate. Then, eat the potential offender, wait 20 minutes, and take your pulse again. If your pulse rate increases more than 10 beats per minute, you have uncovered a possible allergen. Drop the food from your diet, and test again in a month to confirm. During that time, you may notice withdrawal symptoms followed by a greater sense of health.

Specific Nutrients

Dietary deficiencies are often found in people who suffer from arthritis. Blood levels of the following nutrients are often low in individuals with joint pain, and their symptoms improve when supplemented: vitamins C, E, B-3, B-5, and B-6, and the minerals calcium, magnesium, selenium, and zinc. Other nutrients likely play supporting roles as well. I will mention just some that have been studied.

✦ **Vitamin C and vitamin E** Deficiency of vitamin C results in altered collagen synthesis and compromised connective tissue repair. Several studies have reported that vitamin C has a positive effect on cartilage; moreover, cartilage erosion and overall changes in and around the arthritic joints were found to be much less in animals kept on high doses of vitamin C.[17] This same study indicated that vitamin E appears to possess a synergistic action with vitamin C; thus, the researchers concluded that judicious use of these vitamins, either alone or in combination with other therapies, may be of great benefit to people suffering from OA. A clinical trial of vitamin E (600 IU) alone in patients with OA demonstrated that vitamin E was significantly more effective than a placebo in relieving pain.[18]

✦ **Pantothenic acid**   In an older study, megadoses (2 g daily) of pantothenic acid relieved symptoms of RA.[19] Stopping treatment caused symptoms to return. Improvements in OA symptoms have been reported using smaller doses (12.5 mg daily) of pantothenic acid, and although it often took one to two weeks before progress was noted, it did work.[20] Recommended dosages of pantothenic acid range from 15 mg to 2,000 mg per day. Start with the lowest dose only and increase if necessary. Good sources of pantothenic acid include: beef liver, egg, avocado, milk, chicken, peanut butter, bananas, and potatoes. For the precise amount of this nutrient contained in certain foods, consult Appendix C. Because the amounts found naturally in foods are so low, you may need to supplement.

✦ **Niacin (vitamin B-3)**   Niacin has been tested with hundreds of patients and found valuable in treating OA and RA. Since the doses used were in the upper range (4 g) and may cause druglike reactions, it is advisable to take this amount only under medical supervision. Side effects include glucose intolerance and liver damage in sensitive people. Daily doses of up to 1,000 mg of niacin appear to be safe and can be taken in a multivitamin supplement or B-complex tablet. A characteristic flushing of the skin will occur with this dosage of niacin; however, the niacinamide form does not produce this sensation.

✦ **Zinc**   Zinc is a possible contributor to the nutritional treatment of arthritis. Sufferers usually have lower than normal zinc levels in their blood and, when supplemented, show noticeable improvements in morning stiffness, joint swelling, and the patients' own impression of their condition.[21] Zinc, along with vitamin A, B-6, and E and the mineral copper, are required for the synthesis of normal collagen and maintenance of cartilage structure. A deficiency of any one would allow for accelerated joint degeneration. Recommended dosage is 15 to 50 mg daily. Good sources of zinc include: oysters, turkey, lima beans, yogurt, and wheat germ. For the precise amount of this nutrient contained in certain foods, consult Appendix C.

Glucosamine Sulfate

One of the best natural treatments for OA may be glucosamine sulfate, found in high concentration in our joint tissues. It stimulates the manufacture of cartilage components necessary for joint repair and exerts a protective effect against joint destruction. Glucosamine sulfate can be derived from the muscle tissue of lobster, crabs, and mussels.

Numerous double-blind studies have shown that glucosamine sulfate is more effective and better tolerated than the common arthritis pain relievers, the nonsteroidal anti-inflammatory drugs (NSAIDs), like aspirin, Nalfon, Motrin, Advil, Nuprin, Indocin, Naprosyn, Feldene, and Clinoril.[22] These may have significant side effects: damage to the intestinal tract, allergic reactions, easy bleeding and bruising, ringing in the ears, fluid retention, and, in extreme cases, kidney and liver damage. Although NSAIDs are fairly effective in suppressing pain and inflammation, when taken for long periods of time they actually worsen the condition by inhibiting cartilage formation and accelerating cartilage destruction (something not frequently disclosed).[23]

NSAIDs offer temporary relief, but glucosamine sulfate addresses the cause of OA—without contraindications or possible and worrisome drug interactions. The down side is that natural methods invariably take longer to work, and you will have to be patient for a few weeks. You can find glucosamine sulfate at health food stores. The dosage is 500 mg three times a day on an empty stomach. If it upsets your stomach, as some supplements do in sensitive people, take it with meals.

Basic Daily Supplements for Arthritis

Multivitamin and mineral complex (without iron)

Check the B-complex for a range of 50–100 mg

Add vitamins and minerals to total the following:

Calcium:	1,500 mg
Magnesium:	750 mg
Vitamin C plus bioflavenoids:	1,000–2,000 mg; 1–3 times daily
Pantothenic acid:	50–2,000 mg
Vitamin E:	600 IU
Zinc:	15–50 mg

Additional Daily Supplements for Arthritis

Fish oil or EPA capsules:	2–3 capsules
Evening primrose oil:	6–8 capsules
Glucosamine sulfate:	3–4 capsules

Herbs for Arthritis

Feverfew, yucca extract, alfalfa, kelp, black cohosh, celery seed, parsley tea, valerian root, devil's claw tea.

Also Helpful for Arthritis

Exercise to reduce pain and retard joint deterioration (except when in pain).

Drink 1–2 quarts of water daily to hydrate joints.

Rest when in pain.

Take hot tubs and baths for pain relief.

Expose yourself to sunlight for 20 minutes per day to help pain and stiffness.

Part Two

PREPARING FOR THE LATER YEARS

9

HEART DISEASE

Heart disease is by and large a
self-inflicted malady. You don't catch it.
—KENNETH COOPER, M.D., MPH

omen tend to think of heart disease as a men's issue, but it is the leading cause of death for women as well. Heart disease affects more women than the five leading causes of cancer deaths in women combined. While 40,000 women die of breast cancer each year, 250,000 die from heart attacks and another 250,000 succumb to other diseases of the heart and blood vessels.[1] Because women are "protected" by estrogen before menopause, the incidence of heart disease in women trails behind men 10 to 15 years. According to the American Heart Association, one in nine women aged 45 to 64 has some form of heart or blood-vessel disease; this ratio soars to one in three by age 65 and beyond.

Heart attacks may strike older women as frequently as older men, but, women's prospects for a lasting return to normalcy are much gloomier. About 25 percent more women than men die within a year of having a heart attack.[2] This may be because female heart-attack victims are generally older, hence are more likely to experience complications from other illnesses, but this is speculation. Also, women do not respond to treatments prescribed during or after a heart attack as well as do men. For example, the death rate for women undergoing coronary-bypass surgery is twice that of men. Women are less likely to survive angioplasty, a treatment used to remove the plaque in arteries that is obstructing the flow of blood to the heart, and are twice as likely to have a second heart attack.

Women and their doctors often do not take women's heart symptoms seriously. Women overlook the classic signs of a heart attack: chest pains or tightness, heartburn, shortness of breath, numbness or tingling in the arms or jaw, and sweating. Physicians hesitate to act on such symptoms in women and postpone referring them for diagnostic testing, which may be one reason why women don't fare as well in surgery, the disease being more advanced by that time.[3]

WHAT IS HEART DISEASE?

Heart disease is a broad term used to describe many different diseases of the heart and blood vessels. The blood vessels of the heart, also called *coronary arteries*, supply the heart muscles with vital oxygen and nutrients. If the flow of blood is restricted or blocked, severe damage to the heart can occur—the heart attack.

Some thickening and hardening of the arteries, a process called *arteriosclerosis*, is normal. A more insidious and advanced stage, *atherosclerosis*, occurs when the condition accelerates and the artery linings build up to the point of obstruction. The substance responsible for clogging the arteries—made up of fatty material, cholesterol, cellular waste products, calcium, and fibrin—is collectively referred to as *plaque*.

Atherosclerosis doesn't happen overnight, not even at menopause. It is a gradual process that takes almost a lifetime. Preventing the accumulation of plaque must start in the early years, maybe as early as childhood. Even children have been found to have fat deposits in their arteries that may later form into artery-clogging plaque.

HORMONES AND THE HEART

Do hormones promote or prevent cardiovascular disease? It's hard to know. News articles quote studies from prestigious medical journals that seem to contradict each other, creating fear and confusion. Earlier reports agreed that the relatively high levels of estrogen found in the Pill of the 1960s caused a twofold or greater increase in the incidence of heart attacks and strokes. Recent research reverses this stand. A study conducted through the National Institutes of Health showed the death rate from heart disease in women on ERT to be one-third that of a control group of women not taking estrogen.[4] A 10-year follow-up study from the Nurses' Health Study concluded that women who had taken estrogen after menopause were half as likely to develop or die from heart disease.[5]

Whether ERT actually prevents heart disease remains to be proven. Several researchers have suggested that, since the women selected for ERT studies were generally healthier, slimmer, more active, and more health conscious, their reduced risk may have been due to their lifestyle rather than the hormone. Yet, the results are impressive and something to consider if you are at high risk.

Another question nags away at women who are trying to make an informed decision about their future. Does taking a progestin with estrogen (HRT), which is what most midlife women are doing, confer the same protection as estrogen alone? So far, it doesn't seem to. While estrogen increases HDL levels (the good cholesterol) and lowers LDL levels (the bad guys), the hormone progesterone (or progestin, the synthetic version used in HRT) may counter this reaction and thus possibly even *raise* the risk of heart disease. Some studies have, in fact, linked the addition of progestogens to an increase in the risks of heart disease and stroke.[6] Obviously, more studies are needed to provide us with greater assurance that the hormones we take do indeed protect us from heart disease.

Further research is underway to resolve some of these questions. The National Institutes of Health has funded a massive study on health issues unique to women. The Women's Health Initiative will focus primarily on how diet, hormone therapy, calcium, and vitamin D can prevent heart disease, osteoporosis, and cancers of the breast, colon, and rectum. Hopefully in 5 or 10 years we will have a better understanding of HRT. For now, there are many known risk factors and lifestyle characteristics that affect the incidence of coronary heart disease and on which we can take action.

RISK FACTORS FOR HEART DISEASE

Risk factors are traits or habits that make a person more susceptible to disease. Some risk factors for heart-related problems, like age and genetic inheritance, cannot be altered; most are conditions over which we have a great deal of control.

Genetics

The fact that there is a link between families and incidence of heart disease is undeniable; the question remains, is it nature or nurture? Just because heart disease runs in families doesn't necessarily mean that increased risk is genetic in origin, according to researchers at the Center for Inherited Diseases at the University of Washington in Seattle. They found that the wives of their male heart-disease patients also had a greater risk for heart disease, suggesting that the spouses had some of the same unhealthy habits as their sick husbands.[7]

Age

Women tend to manifest heart problems about 10 to 15 years later in life than men, but as mentioned above, by the age of 65 to 74 years, the incidence is the same in both sexes. Also, the older a woman is, the more apt she is to develop high blood pressure and high blood-cholesterol levels, to be diabetic, overweight, and more sedentary—all additional risk factors.

Ethnicity

African American women are 25 percent more likely to die of coronary heart disease than Caucasian women, and their death rate for stroke is 83 percent higher. Hypertension is more common in black women of all ages, and they experience it earlier in life, suffer more severely, and die from hypertension-related causes more frequently. Paying close attention to the lifestyle factors that regulate high blood pressure is crucial for the young black woman.

Cigarettes

Women who smoke are two to six times as likely to suffer a heart attack as nonsmokers, and the risk increases with the number of cigarettes smoked per day.[8] Smoking is more of a risk factor for women than for men; a 55-year-old woman who smokes is in more danger of having a heart attack than a male smoker of the same age.[9] Surprisingly, women in the United States who smoke die almost as often from heart disease as from lung cancer.

Smoking affects the circulatory system in a number of ways. The carbon monoxide in cigarette smoke reduces the blood's oxygen-carrying ability, so less oxygen is available to the heart and other organs. Smoking decreases HDLs and raises LDLs. It damages the lining of the arteries, setting the stage for the development of coronary lesions. Smoking also increases the likelihood of clot formation, irregular heart rhythms, and coronary spasms. And if that's not enough, women who smoke experience menopause an average of two to three years earlier than nonsmokers, which itself is another risk factor for heart disease.

No matter how many years you have smoked, when you quit, your risk of heart disease declines. Within two years of stopping, your chances of a heart attack will be cut in half; 10 years after stopping, your risk of dying from a heart attack will be almost the same as if you never smoked at all.[10]

Most women know this already, but do not take oral contraceptives if you smoke. If you do, your risk of a heart attack escalates 40 times.[11]

Alcohol

The French outlive Americans by about $2\frac{1}{2}$ years and suffer 40 percent fewer heart attacks—despite the fact that smoking is a national pastime and their diet swims in a big pool of fat.[12] This shocking revelation seems to contradict all we have heard and read about heart disease.

Several population studies have suggested that *moderate* amounts of alcohol (one to two drinks per day) may help prevent heart disease. Alcohol appears to help the heart by raising HDLs, decreasing the stickiness of blood platelets, and lowering the levels of fibrinogen, a potent risk factor for heart disease. European researchers have found that red wine contains phenolic compounds, which have strong antioxidant properties that limit the oxidation of LDLs.[13]

Is it wine that wards off heart attacks in the French, or is it because they eat more fresh fruits and vegetables than Americans, take longer to relish their meals, and use more olive oil and less butter in their cooking? In other words, is it because their entire lifestyle is more stress-free than that of the typical American. When headlines sensationalize one food or substance and label it a "cure," it is important to realize that, when it comes to disease and health, many factors participate.

Moderation is the operative word. Heavy drinking, or more than three glasses a day, can reduce blood flow to the heart and upset its rhythm, causing irregular heart beats, raised blood pressure and blood triglyceride levels, and eventually damage to the heart muscle. Some studies suggest a connection between alcohol intake and breast cancer; until we know more, it may be wise to substitute mineral water for wine part of the time. Keep in mind that alcohol provides no nutrition—only extra calories. Women who are trying to control their weight may want to save alcohol, just as they do dessert, for special occasions.

Diabetes

A diabetic woman with heart disease is more at risk for dying of a heart attack than a diabetic man.[14] Total blood cholesterol is frequently higher in diabetic women, and HDL cholesterol lower. Elevated blood-sugar levels also damage the lining of the arterial walls, increasing their vulnerability to plaque formation. Heart disease is just one of the many complications associated with diabetes. Be as diligent as you can about reducing other risk factors if you are diabetic.

Excess Weight

Mildly to moderately overweight midlife women are at up to 40 times the risk of coronary disease as women of normal weight, according to a Harvard University School of Medicine study.[15]

Also, women who gain weight during the middle years are at twice the risk of developing heart disease as women who have been overweight all their lives. The researchers in this study predict that as much as 40 percent of coronary disease in women could be prevented by weight loss alone.

Where you store your extra fat can be an additional hazard. If you thicken up in the waist and abdomen, your risk increases more than if you accumulate fat in the hips and thighs.

Sedentary Living

At the top of the risk factor pyramid, along with cigarette smoking and high-blood cholesterol, is sedentary living. There is a significant relationship between physical inactivity and the risk for coronary heart disease.[16] In 1987, Kenneth Powell and his colleagues from the Centers for Disease Control in Atlanta scrutinized the findings of 40 major studies of this relationship. They concluded that inactivity is as great a risk factor for death from heart disease as any of the better-known factors.

A recent study conducted at the Aerobics Center in Dallas, Texas, shows that even a moderate level of physical activity, such as a brisk walk of 30 to 60 minutes each day, significantly reduces the risk of dying from heart disease.[17] No matter what your age, an active lifestyle and a regular exercise program can keep your heart healthy. Exercise burns fat, thus regulating weight; it raises your protective HDLs and lowers your LDL cholesterol levels; it lowers your blood pressure and your heart rate; and it promotes more efficient use of insulin, which helps control diabetes. If there is a magic pill for heart disease, exercise is it.

Stress

We are all aware of the connection between stress and disease. Years ago many of us read the 1974 bestseller, *"Type A" Behavior and Your Heart*, by Meyer Friedman and Ray Rosenman, and learned how men who have an aggressive "type A" personality are more prone to heart disease. I don't know if this is still considered true for men, but studies on women show no connection between type A behavior and heart disease. Another factor that has been linked to women's stress and increased heart problems is working outside the home. The famous Framingham Heart Study that began in 1948 finds flaws here as well, as no connection appears to exist between heart disease and working in or out of the home.

Even though the exact role stress plays remains unclear, we cannot rule it out as a potential area of concern. Several studies suggest that continued emotional crises that trigger the fight-or-flight response may eventually lead to permanent elevation in blood pressure, heart rate, and blood-cholesterol levels. Whether it is stress itself that is physically harmful, or the *effects* of stress—such as overeating, overdrinking, and being overweight—that stack the cards against us, we must learn how to counter the effects of a stress-filled life. Proven ways to ease tension include exercise, relaxation techniques, yoga, meditation, massages, hot baths, long walks, recreational reading, and movies. Whatever works to relax you may also protect your heart.

Social Isolation and Self-Involvement

Many studies show that people who live alone and have no social network have a higher risk of dying early. A report reviewing several studies found evidence that social isolation heightens people's susceptibility to illness and disease. It suggests that not having someone to share private feelings or have close contact with is as significant a risk factor as all the others we know.[18] Anything that develops intimacy and feelings of connection can be healing in all senses of the word.

People who live alone are prone to self-involvement. Interviews from a nine-year research study involving almost 13,000 men found that the participants who talked more about themselves developed heart disease more often than those who did not.[19] Most striking was the even greater degree of self-involvement of those who ultimately died.

Midlife women often find themselves alone because of divorce or death. Keeping active in social groups, clubs, and other supportive groups may provide more than a fun evening; it may protect the heart.

High Blood Pressure

Elevated blood pressure, also known as *hypertension*, contributes to cardiovascular disease and stroke. Even slight elevations double the risk. High blood pressure is symptomless; you may feel great and not have a clue that it is silently damaging your body. Left untreated, hypertension can lead to kidney disease and vision loss. It is imperative to have your blood pressure checked regularly.

Hypertension refers to a higher than normal force exerted by the blood against the elastic walls of the arteries. The heart generates pressure to pump blood throughout the body, and the muscular arteries contract to help it along. Each time the heart contracts, pressure in the arteries increases; each time the heart relaxes between beats, the pressure drops. Thus, there are two pressures that are measured to evaluate the heart's condition: an upper (systolic) pressure and a lower (diastolic) pressure.

As a general rule, systolic pressure, the first number, falls between 100 and 140, and diastolic pressure falls between 60 and 90. Many charts cite 120/80 as the optimum for a healthy adult, but it is possible to have a different reading and still be quite healthy. By taking several readings over a period of time you can determine what is normal for you.

According to the National Heart and Lung Institute, certain women fall into a higher risk category.[20] Those women most susceptible to heart disease include:

+ older women (more than half of all women over age 55 suffer)

+ women taking the Pill (1 in 20 women who take estrogen have an elevated blood pressure)[21]

+ women near the end of pregnancy (hypertension usually subsides after the birth of the child)

+ nonwhite women (especially African Americans)

Although high blood pressure can rarely be cured, it responds well to lifestyle changes. Good nutrition, exercise, weight control, and relaxation techniques bring blood pressure down safely and effectively. This natural treatment is particularly desirable when you weigh it against the side effects of the common antihypertensive drugs (vasodilators, diuretics, and beta-blockers): depression, heart palpitations, dizziness, muscle spasms, menstrual irregularity, nausea, weakness, dry mouth, mental confusion, insomnia, headaches, drowsiness, nightmares, twitching, loss of sexual desire, rash, and swelling of the breasts.

Women who have adverse reactions to drugs will be encouraged to know that recent studies show that nutritional therapy can substitute for drugs in most cases or, if drugs are still needed, can lessen some side effects.[22]

Natural Treatments for Reducing High Blood Pressure

✦ Lose weight if necessary (overweight women are 2 to 3 times more likely to develop high blood pressure, or HBP)

✦ Decrease chronic stress (repeated stress may temporarily or permanently elevate blood pressure)[23]

✦ Exercise regularly (exercise has a beneficial effect on blood pressure regardless of any change in body weight)

✦ Maintain a low-stress diet (low in salt, sugar, coffee, tea, and saturated fats)

✦ Avoid oral contraceptives, especially if you smoke

✦ Eat foods high in potassium (fresh vegetables, bananas, orange juice, beans, nuts, and molasses)

✦ Supplement daily with the following
   calcium (1,000 mg)
   magnesium (500 mg)
   zinc (30 mg)
   vitamin C (1,000–2,000 mg)
   B-complex (20–50 mg)

✦ Eat garlic (minced in foods or in capsule form)

THE ROLE OF CHOLESTEROL

High levels of cholesterol in the blood contribute to the development of plaque and thus raise one's risk for coronary heart disease. Cholesterol itself is not harmful; on the contrary, it is vital to our existence. It plays multiple roles in our biological functioning: it lines our cells and helps carry out basic functions of life; it insulates the nerves and allows normal transmission of nerve impulses; and it participates in the manufacture of certain hormones and hormone-like vitamins, such as estrogen and vitamin D. We can get cholesterol from food, but our body manufactures all it requires.

Some people confuse cholesterol with fat, yet it really isn't a fat at all, but a lipid: a waxy substance carried in the bloodstream along with several types of fat and proteins. Since fat and water don't mix, the liver combines fat and cholesterol with protein carriers called *lipoproteins*, so they can travel through the blood to be deposited in the cells. Lipoproteins in turn can help prevent or contribute to heart disease.

Total Cholesterol

below 200 mg/dl . . . . . . desirable

200–239 . . . . borderline

240 or above . . . . high risk

LDL Levels

below 130 mg/dl . . . . desirable

130–159 . . . . borderline

160 or above . . . . high risk

HDL Levels

50 mg/dl or above . . . . . desirable

35–50 . . . . borderline

below 35 . . . . high risk

Triglycerides

20–140 mg/dl normal

140–190 . . . . monitor

above 190 . . . . high risk

Ratio of Total Cholesterol to HDL

above 4.5 . . . . desirable

below 4.5 . . . . higher risk

Low-Density Lipoproteins (LDLs)

The chief carriers of cholesterol to the cells are the LDLs, also referred to as the "bad" cholesterol. Their reputation stems from studies showing that a 1-percent greater LDL value is associated with a slightly more than 2-percent increase in coronary artery disease over a six-year period.[24] The higher the LDL levels in the blood, the more cholesterol is available to clog the coronary arteries and bring on atherosclerosis. LDLs remain longer in the bloodstream in some people than in others; the more LDLs there are and the longer they linger, the greater the risk. One reason postmenopausal women are more susceptible to heart disease is that LDL levels rise after menopause.

LDL values are strongly influenced by diet. And here is a clue as to what works: vegetarians have much lower LDL levels than omnivores.

High-Density Lipoproteins (HDLs)

The "good" carriers of cholesterol are called the HDLs. HDLs seem to mobilize cholesterol out of the arteries and carry it to the liver, where it is converted into bile and excreted. People with very low levels of HDLs are more prone to heart attacks: a 1-percent lower HDL value is associated with a 3- to 4-percent increase in coronary artery disease.[25] Even when total cholesterol levels are below 200 mg/dl, decreased HDL levels are associated with a greater incidence of heart attacks in both men and women.

The levels of HDL in the bloodstream are determined partly by your genetic code and partly by lifestyle factors such as weight, exercise, smoking, and diet. Before menopause, women's HDLs are generally higher then men's, and this may account for their lowered incidence of heart disease.

Triglycerides

Triglycerides are fatty substances formed in the liver from the food you eat, and by the body's own synthesis of internal fat, to be used for energy or storage. Some researchers have found that elevated TGs are predictors of heart disease, especially in women over 50. TGs rise with age, are higher in overweight people, and can be increased by taking the Pill and ERT.

Testing for Cholesterol Levels

Women need to be as conscientious about their blood cholesterol as men. For an accurate assessment it is essential that you undergo a blood test to get the complete lipid profile—that is, not just your total cholesterol reading, but the individual levels of HDL, LDL, and TG, and the ratio of HDL to total cholesterol. The most recent data suggest that the total cholesterol-to-HDL ratio is a better measure of risk for coronary heart disease than either total cholesterol or LDL levels.[26]

DIET FOR A HEALTHY HEART

An extensive body of studies, laboratory findings, and clinical evidence has established an association, if not a causative link, between diet and heart disease. For the most part, attention has been focused on fat and fiber intake, although a variety of other foods and a host of nutrients are now known to aggravate or protect against various heart problems.

Fat

Of all the nutritional factors involved in circulatory problems, total dietary fat is the most important. Lower your overall fat intake, and your risk drops markedly. Control saturated fat, and you lower blood cholesterol and your risk even further. The American diet is close to 40 percent fat, a figure that must be cut roughly in half. The exact amount of recommended dietary fat varies from the American Heart Association's upper limit of 30 percent to the bottom-line of 5 to 10 percent advocated by many progressive nutritionists. Many eminent researchers suggest that a heart-healthy diet is one that restricts fat to between 20 to 25 percent of total caloric intake.

Over the last several years there has been exciting news: proof that heart disease can not only be prevented with dietary changes, but can actually be reversed. A well-known study by Dean Ornish, director of the Preventive Medicine Research Institute in Sausalito, California, has shown that in only one year, patients with severe arterial blockages began to unclog when they followed a comprehensive lifestyle program.[27] Better yet, the only known side effects of the program are positive ones.

The Ornish program includes giving up smoking, exercising moderately, following daily stress-management classes, and drastically changing dietary habits. The diet for reversing heart disease is more stringent than one would follow for prevention. It is primarily vegetarian, and consists of 10 percent fats, 15 to 20 percent protein, and up to 75 percent complex carbohydrates. The basic difference between this and a generally healthy food plan is the lowered level of fat, but treating a disease state usually involves some stringent measures. At the end of one year, Ornish's patients showed significant overall reduction of atherosclerosis and coronary heart disease. The program is outlined in his book, *Reversing Heart Disease*.

✦ **Saturated fat**   The worst single dietary offender in heart disease is saturated fat. Saturated fats clog the arteries and raise blood cholesterol levels. They are generally solid at room temperature and come primarily from animal products such as red meat, poultry (especially the skin), whole milk, cheese, butter, and cream. Many people confuse saturated fat with cholesterol. While they may be found together in many animal products, they are different substances. Prime rib contains both saturated fat and cholesterol; lobster is full of cholesterol but has no saturated fat. Which is worse for the heart? Both are thought to raise blood-cholesterol levels, but if there were a contest, saturated fat would win hands down.

A few vegetable oils are also saturated and carry the same risks, even though they do not contain cholesterol. Palm kernal and coconut oil are highly saturated fats—in fact, even more saturated than beef fat. These oils are commonly used by manufacturers in making every snack imaginable, from crackers and chips to cookies, cakes, whipped dessert toppings, and granola bars.

✦ **Trans fatty acids**   Trans fatty acids are found in the margarines, shortenings, and cooking fats used to prepare french fries, corn chips, commercial baked goods, and dozens of other processed products. Using a chemical process called "hydrogenation," naturally occurring oils, such as peanut oil and coconut oil, are converted into saturated fats that are solid at room temperature and do not turn rancid quickly.

Early studies showed they could raise cholesterol levels; recent research from Harvard Medical School has linked them to a higher risk for heart disease. Epidemiologist Walter Willet calculated the intake of trans fatty acids from a questionnaire completed by over 87,000 women as part of the Nurses' Health Study. During the following eight years, 431 of the nurses had heart attacks. Those who consumed the most trans fatty acids had a 50 percent higher rate of heart disease than those who did not.[28] Women who ate margarine four or more times a day had a 66 percent higher risk of heart disease than those who ate it less than once a month.

Food manufacturers are not currently required to list the amounts of trans fatty acids in their products, so there is no way of knowing how much is hidden in the items you buy. Check labels for "partially hydrogenated vegetable oils." If they are one of the first three ingredients listed, you can be certain you are getting a high-fat food. A quick measure for total fats is that if the product has more than 3 grams of fat per 100 calories, it's over the 30-percent limit. The main point is that we must minimize both saturated fats and trans fatty acids in our diets.

✦ **Polyunsaturated fats**   Polyunsaturated fats, generally liquid at room temperature, are derived from vegetable sources such as corn, safflower, and soybean. Most vegetable oils, except for coconut and palm oils, are not saturated, and have been shown to lower blood cholesterol levels. Evidence is mounting, however, that these fats may lower the "good" as well as the "bad" cholesterol and may also be implicated in the development of breast cancer. Although the research is still speculative, there are enough data to recommend substituting for these oils as well with the oils considered safest to eat, the monounsaturated fats.

✦ **Monounsaturated oils**   The Greeks and Italians thrive on a diet low in saturated fats and plentiful in both complex carbohydrates and monounsaturated oils. The fact that inhabitants of these countries suffer half as many fatal heart attacks as we in the United States is thought to be due to their fondness for olive oil, but we cannot forget that more than one factor may be producing such heart-healthy people. A diet rich in monounsaturated oils like olive oil, peanut oil, and canola oil makes LDLs more resistant to oxidation than a diet high in polyunsaturated oils like corn and most other vegetable oils.[29] This is a plus, because oxidized fats may be potent artery cloggers. If your recipe calls for oil, go for the monounsaturates.

✦ **Fish oils** The health benefits of fish oils have been widely investigated since it became known that Eskimos have a low incidence of heart disease despite their traditional diet of whale and seal fat. Further studies noted that the Japanese also have a diet rich in fish and show a similarly reduced rate of heart disease. In 1985, after 20 years of following a group of men, scientists from the Netherlands concluded that there was in fact an inverse relationship between fish consumption and death from coronary artery disease and that as little as one or two fish dishes a week may be valuable for prevention.[30]

Fish and fish oils, which are omega-3 fatty acids, have been ascribed a broad spectrum of biological benefits. They are reported to lower blood pressure, reduce blood lipids, and improve blood flow and prevent blood platelets (which aid in blood clotting) from forming. As platelet inhibitors they may even be more effective than aspirin, the most common agent thus far.[31]

The active ingredients of fish oils are eichosapentaenoic acid (EPA) and docosahexaenoic acid (DHA). EPA originates in plants and algae; fish eat them and store the EPA in their muscles and liver. No food sources of EPA in a vegetarian diet can match the concentration in fish. The best fish sources are high fat fish such as salmon, mackerel, sablefish, Florida pompano, bluefin tuna, swordfish, bluefish, shark, and herring. If you do not regularly eat fish, you can supplement with 1,000 to 3,000 mg of EPA or omega-3 fatty acid capsules several times a week.

Fiber

There is strong evidence that oat bran and other foods high in soluble fiber can lower blood cholesterol. An analysis of 20 studies concluded that approximately 3 grams of soluble fiber per day from oat products can lower the total cholesterol level 5 to 6 mg/dl, and that the reduction is greater in those with initially high blood-cholesterol levels.[32] Oat bran should not be used to replace a low-fat

Sources of Oat Bran

OAT SOURCE	GRAMS OF OAT BRAN
oat bran (1 Tbsp.)	15
oat bran muffin (1)	10–15
oat bran cereal (1 oz.)	4–5
oatbran bread (1 slice)	2.5–3

diet but in addition to one. You should also be aware that many of the oat muffins and crackers on the market are swimming in fat that negates any cholesterol-lowering effect of the bran.

Nature has provided us with a wide variety of fibrous foods: black-eyed peas; kidney, navy, lima, and pinto beans; carrots; green peas; corn; prunes; sweet potatoes; zucchini; bananas; apples; pears; and oranges are some of the best. If you like these foods anyway, add them to your daily menu and lower your cholesterol levels.

Supplemental fiber is an effective way to lower blood-cholesterol levels when total dietary intake is low or dietary modification is not working. A supplement containing 4 grams of guar gum and 3.5 grams of pectin mixed with three types of insoluble fiber was given to patients with a history of mild to high cholesterol. After 15 weeks, total cholesterol, LDL, and the ratio of LDL to HDL were significantly reduced.[33] Other kinds of supplemental fiber proved equally beneficial. Daily dietary supplements of 15 grams of grapefruit pectin significantly lowered plasma cholesterol and improved LDL to HDL ratio in patients with high cholesterol levels who were unable or unwilling to follow a low-risk diet.[34] Adding 7.3 grams of psyllium, an edible fibrous seed, to cereal reduced total serum cholesterol concentration after two weeks.[35] I would not recommend fiber supplementation as your first line of defense, but as an adjunct to a broader program it can prove useful.

Soy Protein

Although animal protein promotes elevated cholesterol, plant protein many inhibit or reduce cholesterol synthesis in the liver. Soy protein, in particular, helps maintain strong arterial walls and promotes resorption of plaque that builds up in the coronary arteries.[35] Soy proteins are part of a group of plant chemicals called *phytosterols* that have the ability to inhibit the absorption of cholesterol, thus keeping down cholesterol levels in the blood.

There is no current recommendation for optimum amounts of phytosterol foods. However, incorporating more plant hormones into your diet may benefit your blood-lipid profile. Tofu, a power-packed phytosterol, can easily replace the meat in burgers, sandwiches, and burritos. It also tastes great with vegetables and can replace cheese in casseroles, burritos, enchiladas, and lasagna.

ANTIOXIDANTS

One of the most important recent discoveries in nutrition and aging research is that oxygen, our basic source of energy and life, has a dark side. At the molecular level, oxygen can form highly reactive biochemical compounds, called *free radicals*. When not tempered by antioxidants, free radicals can start branching chain reactions that reproduce uncontrollably, attacking the cells in the body, destroying cell membranes, and contributing to accelerated aging and age-related diseases. Some of the conditions studied so far that may be related to damage from free radicals are cancer, heart disease, emphysema, rheumatoid arthritis, and Parkinson's disease.[16]

Oxidation is triggered by environmental pollutants as well as by our metabolism. We are bombarded with influences from the outside and from substances we absorb—ultraviolet light, radiation (including X-rays), air pollution, cigarette smoke, pesticides, alcohol, rancid fats—that promote free-radical activation and cellular damage. Many of the external influences are beyond our control, but not all.

The body houses a complex antioxidant system composed of enzymes, vitamins, and minerals, which neutralize free radicals before they damage tissues. These self-manufactured and food-derived antioxidants may or may not serve us adequately, depending on a number of factors, such as what we eat and whether we smoke or drink alcohol. By middle age our ability to maintain this defense system declines, and the antioxidants we obtain from food cannot make up for the lack in our system. By resupplying the body with the full range of antioxidants we may be able to safeguard against the diseases of aging.

Antioxidants have hit the media with a bang. Television commercials and magazine advertisements extol the benefits of these miracle nutrients—but what exactly are they? Antioxidants have been used commercially for years. The food industry adds synthetic antioxidants like BHT and BHA, or the vitamins C and E, to cooking oils and canned meats to prevent the fats in them from oxidizing and turning rancid. The use of antioxidants to prevent aging and disease is a relatively novel concept, however, though research does go back several decades. Below are explanations of the antioxidants, what they do, where to find them food sources, and how much of them we need.

Vitamin E

Vitamin E, along with other antioxidants such as vitamin C, beta carotene, and selenium, are being acclaimed as protectors of the body's cells. Individually and collectively, they appear to help specifically by preventing oxidation of LDL, thereby inhibiting the formation of plaque and the destruction of the blood-vessel linings. The susceptibility of LDL to oxidation is inversely related to the presence of antioxidants in the blood, most notably, vitamin E. In simpler terms: when vitamin E intake is high, LDL and the risk of heart disease is lowered. Many studies confirm that low vitamin E intake is a better predictor of heart disease than elevated cholesterol levels.

Two large-scale studies, one of men and one of women, have shown that large doses of vitamin E (100 IU) lower the risk of heart disease. The more than 80,000 women studied were followed for eight years. Both studies found that vitamin E, when obtained only through diet or even when supplemented as a basic multivitamin and mineral tablet, offered little or no protection; therapeutic doses were needed for a protective effect.[38]

Vitamin E is most known for its antioxidant role, but it also protects the heart by inhibiting platelet formation. In one test, after two weeks of 200 IU of vitamin E, platelet adhesion was reduced by 75 percent; after two weeks of 400 IU, platelet adhesion was reduced 82 percent.[37] Researchers noted that the inhibitory activity of alpha-tocopherol (our main form of vitamin E) was dose-dependent; higher doses offered greater benefits. You should supplement if you feel you are at high risk for heart disease, or if you just want the best possible protection. Good sources of vitamin E include: sunflower seeds, almonds, crab, sweet potatoes, vegetable oils, fish, and wheat germ. For the precise amount of this nutrient contained in certain foods, consult Appendix C.

Vitamin C

In a study of both men and women, it was found that high levels of vitamin C concentration in the blood may lower the risk for heart disease.[39] The researchers concluded that even in a well-nourished population with perfectly adequate concentrations of plasma vitamin C at intakes well above the RDA of 60 mg, there is still an association between vitamin C levels and HDL. What this means is that the RDA levels are not enough to result in antioxidizing effects.

The Nurses' Health Study, which examined 87,000 women between 34 and 54 years of age, found the risk of developing heart disease was more than 42 percent lower for women who took high doses of vitamin C as compared with women with low vitamin C intakes. Sources of vitamin C include: raw green peppers, orange juice, broccoli, cantaloupe, strawberries, fresh tomato, and potatoes. For the precise amount of this nutrient contained in certain foods, consult Appendix C.

Beta Carotene

Researchers at Harvard Medical School set out to study the relationship between beta carotene and cancer, and whether aspirin had any protective effect against heart disease. Surprisingly, they found that in the men taking beta carotene, incidences of heart disease and strokes were cut in half.[40] Another recent study found that beta carotene, along with vitamin E, can reduce the risk of a first heart attack.[41] Individually, but even better collectively, antioxidants have been proven to guard against this killer, and many more studies concerning the roles and benefits of antioxidants are in progress.

The recommended dosage for beta carotene as an antioxidant ranges between 15 to 50 mg per day and can be met with less effort than some of the other antioxidants. Good sources of beta carotene include: spinach, carrots, sweet potatoes, winter squash, cantaloupe, and broccoli.

Selenium

Selenium is another vital antioxidant that protects cell membranes from damage by highly reactive oxygen fragments. Regional studies on the incidence of cardiovascular disease and soil levels of selenium show a higher rate of heart attacks and stroke in areas of the United States where soil is low in selenium.[42] The so-called "stroke-belt" in Georgia and the Carolinas are areas of very low selenium soil content and correspondingly the highest levels of heart disease and stroke in the country.

There is sufficient reason to supplement the diet with 50 to 200 mcg of selenium daily as a protection against heart disease. Many researchers prefer the organic forms, derived from a special type of brewer's yeast, to the inorganic sodium selenite. Inorganic selenium cannot be taken with vitamin C because it decreases its absorption; it has also been reported to be toxic at high levels when taken for a long time. Neither is true of organic selenium. Because of its synergistic effects with vitamin E, it is good to take them together as part of a multivitamin and mineral formula.

The selenium content of food is dependent on the amount found in the soil in which the food was grown and can vary as much as 200-fold. Grains such as whole wheat, brown rice, and oatmeal are fairly good sources if the soil is rich in selenium. Meats, poultry, and fish contain higher amounts, but these may not be preferred sources for many people. Good sources of selenium include: lobster, tuna, shrimp, ham, eggs, chicken, whole wheat bread, and whole grain cereal. For the precise amount of this nutrient contained in certain foods, consult Appendix C.

B VITAMINS

The antioxidants may have to share the spotlight with the B vitamins, which play an entirely different role but are potentially just as important in reducing cardiovascular risk. In the absence of vitamins B-6, B-12, and folic acid, the amino acid *methionine* is converted to a substance known as *homocysteine*. There is convincing proof that an elevated homocysteine level is an independent risk factor for vascular diseases. (Homoscysteine appears to be elevated in postmenopausal women).[43] Several investigators have demonstrated that homocysteine can be normalized with supplementation of these three B vitamins.[44]

DHEA

DHEA (dehydroepiandosterone), a steroid hormone produced by the adrenal glands, can be converted to other hormones such as estrogen, progesterone, and testosterone. Accumulating research suggests that DHEA may be of value in preventing and treating many diseases, including heart disease, cancer, diabetes, obesity, and AIDS. Several studies show that DHEA concentration is inversely related to death from any cause and death from coronary vascular disease in particular.[45] A recent study of heart patients found that a reduced blood level of DHEA is a specific and independent indicator of heart disease.[46]

Dr. Julian Whitaker strongly suggests that people at high risk for heart disease have their DHEA levels measured along with the lipid profile. If they fall below average for their age, they should supplement with DHEA. The dosage for women is 25 to 50 mg per day; for men, 50 to 100 mg per day.[47]

Daily Supplements for a Healthy Heart

✦ Beta carotene (vitamin A)   30 mg
    cuts heart disease and strokes in half

✦ Vitamins B-6, B-12, and folic acid   50 mg
    deficiency raises homocysteine, which
    has a toxic effect on arterial cells

✦ Vitamin C   2,000–3000 mg

✦ Vitamin E   100–400 IU
    increases HDL cholesterol and
    decreases risk of heart disease

◆ Selenium   200 mcg
    a protective antioxidant

◆ Calcium   1,000 mg
    reduces high blood pressure

◆ Magnesium   500 mg
    reduces high blood pressure, and lowers
    the incidence of arrhythmia and sudden
    death by more than 50%

◆ Chromium (picolinate)   200 mcg
    lowers total cholesterol and raises HDLs

◆ Lecithin   2–3 Tbsps.
    lowers cholesterol, reduces triglycerides,
    and raises HDLs

◆ Omega-3 fatty acids   1 g
    increases HDLs and lowers TGs

◆ Garlic   1 clove or
    reduces total cholesterol   2 capsules

◆ L-carnitine   2,000 mg
    reduces angina pain

◆ DHEA   25–50 mg
    decreases risk of heart disease

10

BREAST CANCER

Health is the state about which
medicine has nothing to say.
—W. H. AUDEN

There is no disease that women fear as much as breast cancer—and justifiably so. Breast cancer has become the leading cause of death among women between the ages of 32 and 52. Statistics tell us that the rate of breast cancer has increased 20 percent in the last 20 years, striking one out of eight women. Every 3 minutes a woman is diagnosed, and every 11 minutes a woman dies from the disease.[1] Approximately 80 percent of all breast cancers occur in postmenopausal women, and these rates continue to rise. At one time white women were at a higher risk than African American women, but this has changed; the rates for blacks have doubled, so the incidence is now higher than that in young Caucasian women.

Despite these alarming numbers, we still do not know much about this devastating disease. Despite all the media attention, breast cancer remains an enigma because research on women's health issues has been grossly neglected. All the large or long-term studies on heart disease, cancer, and other major health issues have been conducted exclusively on men. Fortunately, research projects for women have recently been funded, and in the future our children will benefit.

THE RISKS OF HRT

The question most on women's minds when it comes to deciding whether to take hormones is, will they cause breast cancer? The answer isn't clear-cut, but there is enough evidence to warrant concern. When the studies of the estrogen–breast cancer link were collectively examined, researchers calculated that the risk of breast cancer increased with use: the more years a woman was on hormones, the greater the risk. After 15 years on estrogen, they cited a 30-percent increase in breast cancer.[2] HRT appears to be riskier than estrogen alone.[3] And women with a family history of breast cancer who have taken postmenopausal hormones have a twofold greater risk than women who have never taken them.[4]

Many women are not told that hormone treatment can be used shortterm. If you have severe hot flashes and other symptoms but are afraid of the breast-cancer risk, you can opt to use hormones temporarily while learning about other, more natural treatments.

Some forms of ERT may be safer than others. There are actually three forms of estrogen active in the female: estradiol, estrone, and estriol. *Estradiol* is the primary estrogen produced by the ovary. It is converted into the weaker form of *estrone* and then to its weakest dilution, *estriol*. Estradiol and estrone are thought to be the estrogens primarily responsible for facilitating breast cancer. Estriol not only does not stimulate breast tissue growth, it is actually protective against breast cancer.[5]

The most prescribed type of estrogen is conjugated equine estrogen, a mixture of estrogens that come from the urine of pregnant mares, which is converted in the intestinal tract to estrone. The safer version of estrogen, estriol, can also be manufactured for hormone therapy but is not as popular. However, some prominent physicians and cancer specialists are offering what they believe is a safer version of ERT to their patients: a combination of 80 percent estriol, 10 percent estrone, and 10 percent estradiol. This formula is not patented and can be compounded by any pharmacy at your doctor's request. See the *Resources* section at the end of the book for more information on potentially safer forms of hormonal therapy.

My philosophy is: if you don't have symptoms, don't take drugs. When you need relief, first try natural methods; if they fail, seek a health practitioner. If medication is required, try to take something with the fewest side effects, start with the lowest dose, and take it for the shortest amount of time possible. We must participate in our own health and work with our doctors for the program that best fits our needs—for the long term.

RISK FACTORS

Being aware of the risks that predispose you to any disease can save your life if you use that information to take aggressive precautionary measures. It is estimated that about 30 percent of women who develop breast cancer have at least one of the following risk factors. However, it is the 70 percent of women who do *not* identify themselves as potential cancer victims that concern me: they may harbor a false sense of security. It is important for all women to learn how best to protect their bodies.

Risk Factors for Breast Cancer

+ *Heredity:* Risk is greater for those whose mothers, aunts, or sisters have had it.

+ *Age:* Older women are more at risk.

+ *Country of birth:* North American and Northern European women have increased risk.

+ *Socioeconomic class:* Higher-income families have increased risk.

+ *Marital status:* Never-married women have higher risk.

+ *Menarche:* Early menarche (under 12 years) increases risk.

+ *Menopause:* Late menopause (over 55 years) increases risk.

+ *Childbearing experience:* Having had no children or having a first child after 30 increases risk.

+ *Weight:* Being overweight increases risk.

+ *Shape:* Having extra weight distributed in the upper body and stomach, rather than in the hips and thighs, increases risk.

+ *Diet:* A poor diet (high fat, low fiber, low intake of vitamins A, E, C, and selenium) increases risk.

When a disease is as mysterious as cancer and has so many risk factors, we may freeze at the seemingly impossible task of prevention. It is true that a variety of things we eat, breathe, and come into contact with have carcinogenic (cancer-causing) potential. It has been estimated that 90 percent of all cancers are environmentally caused. The good news is, we can identify many of those potentially harmful substances and thus adopt some safeguards to keep cancer from invading our bodies.

DIET

One of the breakthroughs of the 1980s was the finding that diet leads other factors in beating cancer. There are now hard data to prove that specific nutrients can appreciably lower cancer risk.

The conservative American Dietetic Association estimates that 30 to 60 percent of all cancer is nutrition related.[6] Most of the support for these findings comes from years of population studies. Scientists have long suspected a link as they observed that countries in which people primarily eat a high-fat diet—such as the United States, the United Kingdom, and the Netherlands—suffer the world's highest rates of breast cancer, while countries with leaner diets—such as Japan, Thailand, and Poland—have much lower rates. At one time heredity was thought to explain this difference, but the data have since proved otherwise. A landmark 1973 study conducted by a division of the National Cancer Institutes showed that second-generation Japanese women who had lived in California all their lives had breast cancer rates similar to European Americans. Studies from other many countries reach the same conclusion.

Research shows that eating properly may help to prevent breast cancer, and may make the cancer more amenable to treatment if it does occur. According to Sherwood Gorbach, a researcher at Tufts University School of Medicine in Boston, all other risk factors taken together do not appear to have anywhere near the importance of lifestyle factors such as diet.

The evidence is indisputable: poor diet is a major contributor to cancer. Henry Dreher, former senior writer at the Cancer Research Institute, states, "Scientists from the National Academy of Sciences, the National Cancer Institutes, and the American Cancer Society now estimate that 35 percent of all cancers are directly related to diet and the rest may be influenced by it."[7]

The diet that experts now agree will reduce the risk of breast cancer can also reduce the risk of heart disease—and probably many other disease states as well. It is the diet that many nutritionists have advocated for years as the foundation for basic healthy living: eat foods that are low in fat and high in fiber, and supplement when you are lacking in any nutrients.

If you are seriously concerned about breast cancer because you have several risk factors, or if you want to ensure optimum health, there are precautions you can take. Paying attention to the specific types of fat and fiber you eat and incorporating anticancer nutrients in your program can provide protection from cancer in general and breast cancer in particular.

Fat

In 1988 the U.S. government identified limiting excess fat intake as the number one dietary priority of the nation. The Committee on Diet, Nutrition, and Cancer states that, of all the dietary factors studied so far, the evidence is strongest for a causal relationship between fat intake and the occurrence of cancer.[8] The cancers most directly related to a high-fat diet are breast, prostate, colon, and rectal cancer, and the evidence continues to indicate that long-term adherence to a low-fat diet can reduce the risk of several common cancers.[9]

Maureen Henderson, head of the Cancer Prevention Research Program at the Fred Hutchinson Cancer Research Center in Seattle, estimates that if every woman would cut her fat intake in half, breast cancer would drop by as much as 60 percent. Americans now consume an average of 37 percent of their total calories in the form of fat. You may hear that experts recommend total fat intake be around 30 percent of total calories. Even cutting down

to this level is an improvement for most people; however, to reduce the risk of breast cancer, the threshold for results is closer to
20 percent.[10]

Figuring out how much fat you eat is not too difficult, with
all the new books listing fat grams in common foods and the new
food labeling guidelines for packaged products. If you know approximately how many calories you consume in a day, multiply
that number by 0.20 for the optimum total fat calorie count. To
arrive at the optimum number of fat grams, divide your answer by
9 (there are 9 calories in 1 gram of fat). Record what you eat for a
week to get an idea of how much fat you actually are eating. The
comparison of your optimum fat-gram intake to your actual intake
may surprise you.

Example: 2,000 calories x .20 = 400 calories from fat
400/9 = 44 fat grams per day

Fat appears to promote breast cancer in several ways. Studies
consistently show that fatty diets enhance cancerous tumors,
whether they are chemically induced or occur spontaneously. Fat
itself is not thought to be the initiator or carcinogen; rather, excess
fat promotes cancerous growth in cells that are, for whatever reason, predisposed.

Fat is also known to facilitate the growth of breast cancer
through its effect on female hormones. Obesity is clearly associated
with a higher risk of breast, ovarian, and uterine cancer. It is well
established that a high-fat diet, as well as an overfat body, can
increase the production of estrogen, thereby overstimulating the
breast tissue; this can, in turn, result in cancer.

Women must cut their total fat intake. Not only will this
contribute to their overall health and lower their risk for disease, it
will also enable them to lose weight without going on dangerous
starvation diets. The latest approach to weight loss is to minimize
total fat in the diet. It works because it allows you to eat more
food: you are not hungry, you are more satisfied, and you are more
likely to succeed.

A Cornell University study showed that if you choose lean
foods, you can eat relatively large quantities and still lose fat. In

that study a group of women switched from their normal diets to one that had roughly 22 percent of total calories from fat, and they steadily lost about one-half pound a week. This may not sound appealing to women who want to take off ten pounds by Saturday night, but the latest research clearly emphasizes that slower, less dramatic weight loss is healthier. It may interest you to know that the Cornell group did not live on cottage cheese and celery. They ate freely of fruits, vegetables, breads, beans, cereals, pastas, nonfat milk products, lean meats, pretzels, angel-food cake, air-popped popcorn, graham crackers, sherbets, and all the new fat-free desserts.

All fats are not created equal. In premenopausal women, high intakes of animal protein and red meat are associated with increased risk of cancer. For years we have been told to avoid saturated fats—those found in meats, cheeses, and butter—because they are linked to high cholesterol levels and, therefore, to heart disease. Well, guess what? Breast cancer is also associated with a diet high in saturated fat.[11]

Saturated fats are not the only fats to avoid. Vegetable oils that have been transformed into margarine and shortening are no better for you. The process of hydrogenation that converts the oils to solids creates trans fatty acids, and they too cause damage to cells and potentially promote disease. You can find hydrogenated and partially hydrogenated fats in cookies, pies, cakes, french fries, chips, crackers, and dozens of other packaged foods. Check your labels.

A fear of fat can foster some unhealthy reactions too. Not all fats need to be avoided. Our bodies need certain types and amounts of fat to remain healthy. Essential fatty acids, fats that the body cannot make, are needed for the functioning of nerve cells, cellular membranes, and hormone-like substances known as prostaglandins.

Most vegetable oils supply EFAs, and some of these have even been found to promote anticancer activity. Flaxseed oil, for example, is rich in omega-3 fatty acids, which are documented to inhibit tumor production and protect against breast cancer.[12] Other good sources of EFAs are fresh pumpkin seeds, soybean oil, walnut oil, canola oil, wheat germ oil, and fish oils. Increasing fish in your diet also appears to protect against breast cancer. A study involving 26 countries found an increase in fish consumption was associated with lower breast cancer rates.[13] Your best choices are: salmon, mackerel, Florida pompano, herring, bluefish, bluefin tuna, swordfish, and shark.

Fiber

Adding foods high in fiber to your diet may be the second-best precaution you can take against breast cancer. Until recently, research on the role of fiber in relation to cancer had focused on colon cancer, because dietary fiber comes into direct contact with the lining of the digestive tract. Now the benefits of fiber have been shown to extend to breast and other types of cancer too.

Since the 1980s, studies have explored a possible fiber–breast cancer link. Particularly noteworthy is the observation that Finnish women, who consume as much fat as American women but significantly more fiber, have only two thirds the incidence of breast cancer.

Experimental evidence has further confirmed the important role of fiber in prevention of breast cancer. In a recent study conducted by the American Health Foundation in New York, female rats on a high-fat, high-fiber diet were found to be one-third less likely to succumb to breast cancer from a drug-induced breast tumor than those on a high-fat diet alone.[14]

The amount of fiber a woman eats appears to play a part in regulating her estrogen level. Fiber enhances estrogen excretion, which means less of the hormone is reabsorbed into the bloodstream. Thus, the woman's breast tissue is exposed to lower amounts of estrogen. Fiber may also reduce the absorption of fat into the body, thereby also reducing estrogen production. A third possibility is that fiber may bind with and dispose of other carcinogens, keeping them from entering the bloodstream.

Fiber comes in two primary forms: soluble and insoluble. The insoluble, or undigested, form fights cancer better. Health educators have told us for years that insoluble fiber prevents and treats constipation by sweeping food through the intestinal tract. What has not received publicity is the relationship between constipation and breast cancer. If it were a more acceptable topic of conversation, we would probably place greater stress on the necessity of regular bowel movements. Constipation can be a serious health risk. Women who have two or fewer bowel movements a week have four times the incidence of breast disease as women who have one or more movements a day.[15]

Insoluble dietary fiber is found in large quantities in bran and whole grains, and in smaller amounts in fruits and vegetables. The National Cancer Institute recommends that Americans eat up to 30 grams a day; other groups go as high as 40 grams a day. This is more than double what most women currently consume. Make it a priority to figure your fiber intake for a few days to see how close you get to the goal. (See Chapter 15 for a list of fiber foods that fight cancer.)

Antioxidants

Antioxidant nutrients from fresh fruits and leafy green and yellow vegetables have been associated with a reduced risk for many cancers, including breast cancer. Unfortunately, most American women don't eat the recommended four to five servings per day, so supplementation is essential. Supplementing even in low doses can reduce your risk of cancer. In a major study of 15,000 adults in China, a daily dose of antioxidant consisting of 15 mg of beta carotene, 30 mg of vitamin E, and 50 mg of selenium over a five-year period resulted in a 13-percent reduction in total cancer rate.[16]

For over a decade pioneer nutritionists have been advocating the use of supplementation, and within the last few years mainstream health practitioners have come out and publicly admitted that it may be a good idea to take additional antioxidants. The first public health organization to officially recommend vitamin supplements for warding off illnesses such as heart disease and cancer is the Washington, D.C. advocacy group called the Alliance for Aging Research. They advise Americans to take the following: beta carotene, 15–30 mg or 17,000–50,000 IU; vitamin C, 250–1,000 mg; vitamin E, 100–400 IU.[17]

Vitamin A (Beta Carotene)

No other nutrient has captured the attention of cancer researchers the way vitamin A or its precursor, beta carotene, has. Once thought to be effective because it was converted to vitamin A in the body, current research suggests that beta carotene has an independent role as an antioxidant.

Studies in the United States and England note a direct relationship between vitamin A and cancer rates.[18] At least 70 clinical studies have found that people who do not eat fruits and vegetables (which are high in beta carotene and other antioxidants) have a greater incidence of cancer. Scientists leave no doubt that low beta carotene states are associated with an increase in overall cancer death.[19]

Vitamin A requires caution when taken in supplement form, because it can be toxic in large doses. Beta carotene, however, shows no apparent toxicity, even when used in high doses for therapeutic treatment of medical conditions. What is needed is absorbed, and what is not is excreted. The only hazard associated with taking too much beta carotene is an orange tint to the skin. The color may clash with your outfit, but it is not harmful and will wear off after the dosage is lowered.

No RDA has yet been established for beta carotene. A safe daily range is between 15 to 30 mg, or 17,000 to 50,000 IU. It is always a good idea to get what you can from food sources before adding supplements. This is easier for beta carotene, than for some of the other nutrients, and good sources of beta carotene include: spinach, carrots, sweet potatoes, winter squash, cantaloupe, and broccoli. For the precise amount of this nutrient contained in certain foods, consult Appendix C.

Vitamin C

Vitamin C is another powerful antioxidant that blocks free-radical damage. It is also a general detoxifier (removes body toxins or poisons) and is a crucial anticarcinogen. Specifically, it prevents the formation of nitrosamines, potent carcinogens formed from nitrates and nitrites that are found in smoked, pickled, and salt-cured meats.

As with beta carotene, low intakes of vitamin C are associated with increased cancer risk.[20] While no tests have looked directly at vitamin C and breast cancer, factors initiating one type of cancer may be associated with other cancers as well. Studies indicate a strong protective effect of vitamin C for non-hormone-dependent cancers. And an analysis of 46 studies found that in 33 there was a statistically significant degree of protection with high intakes of vitamin C, approximately twice that of a low intake of the vitamin.[21] Researchers also report strong evidence that vitamin C is beneficial in breast cancer prevention.

How much vitamin C is enough to protect the body from disease without exceeding toxic limits? Reviews on the safety of vitamin C fill the literature. At the high end are those who support extreme doses, up to 10,000 mg daily. Therapeutic doses of this magnitude are indicated for some conditions; however, when we are discussing preventive measures and relatively healthy individuals, the dosage need not reach the ceiling. You may want to experiment with amounts by taking up to 5,000 mg (the upper limit of the safety range) and noticing when your stools turn watery. Richard Cathcart, a noted vitamin C expert, came up with the concept of *bowel tolerance*. He feels that if your body needs vitamin C it will absorb it; if not, the excess will be excreted. Some people may stop at 100 mg, some at 6,000 mg. Good sources of vitamin C include: raw green peppers, orange juice, broccoli, cantaloupe, strawberries, potato, and raw tomato. For the precise amount of this nutrient contained in certain foods, consult Appendix C.

Vitamin E

Vitamin E has been under study for several years as a major antioxidant. It is especially effective in blocking the free-radical formation that comes from the oxidation of fats.[22] The process by which fatty foods and oils turn rancid in the presence of oxygen is thought to be a prime contributing cause of breast and colon cancer, and vitamin E is seen as a major ally against it. In addition to its role as a free-radical scavenger, vitamin E enhances the body's immune response and inhibits the conversion of nitrates to the cancer-producing nitrosamines.

Most data support the hypothesis that dietary vitamin E protects against cancer. Women with low blood levels of vitamin E have a much higher risk for breast cancer. In one study, blood levels of vitamin E were correlated with cancer incidence. The analysis revealed that individuals with low levels of vitamin E had about 1.5 times the risk of those who had a higher blood concentration.[23] In a 14-year study of more than 5,000 women in the United Kingdom, low levels of vitamin E were found to increase the incidence of breast cancer by 500 percent.[24]

A reasonable and safe amount of vitamin E for optimum protection is between 400 and 600 IU daily. For those of you concerned with vitamin toxicity, a comprehensive review of the literature states that vitamin E is safe in doses up to 3,000 IU per day.[25] A word of caution for people with special problems: vitamin E intake should always be monitored by a physician if you are taking an anticlotting drug or if you have high blood pressure, liver disease, bilary tract obstruction, or malabsorption syndrome. Good sources of vitamin E include: sunflower seeds, almonds, crab, sweet potatoes, fish, and wheat germ. For the precise amount of this nutrient contained in certain foods, consult Appendix C.

Selenium

Vitamin E works best to prevent cancer when it is teamed with the mineral selenium. Together they are part of a potent anticancer enzyme system that wipes out renegade free radicals. When researchers in Finland examined cancer patients, they found that low levels of selenium increased the risk for cancer, but low selenium plus low vitamin E levels increased the risk even more.[26] More than 55 different studies conducted in 18 countries show the higher the selenium intake, the lower the incidence of breast, colon, and prostate cancer.[27] The National Academy of Sciences has recommended 50 to 200 mcg of selenium daily as a safe range. However, many other scientists feel this level is too low to offer protection. Professors at Cornell University in New York suggest 600 mcg as offering safe but greater protection.[28] When choosing supplemental selenium, look for an organic form as it is better absorbed and less likely to cause toxicity than the inorganic sodium selenite form. Good sources of selenium include: lobster, tuna, shrimp, fish, ham, eggs, chicken, and whole grain bread. For the precise amount of this nutrient contained in certain foods, consult Appendix C.

Other Anticancer Foods

That we should eat a variety of foods is good basic nutritional advice. Although specific nutrients have been singled out and studied in cancer prevention, other foods with unknown properties have also demonstrated cancer-fighting qualities. For example, *cruciferous* vegetables, a unique group of vegetables from the cabbage family, appear to inhibit the formation of cancer cells. These foods contain both sulfur and indoles, substances thought to deactivate carcinogens and protect against cell destruction. Cruciferous vegetables include broccoli, brussels sprouts, cauliflower, and cabbage.

The overwhelming protective effects of fruits and vegetables reported in the literature have aroused interest among scientists who are trying to identify the specific properties in these and other food sources that may guard against cancer. The most recent target for investigation is soy products. After studies with animals indicated a significant inverse relationship between mammary tumors and soybeans, the National Cancer Institute sponsored a workshop to examine the role of soy in reducing cancer risk. The consensus of the workshop was that there are sufficient data to justify further studies.

Soybean consumption is thought to be one of the primary reasons for the relatively low rates of breast cancer in Japan and China. In a case-controlled study of diet and breast cancer among Singapore Chinese, it was found that soy protein had a protective effect.[29] Beta carotene was also found protective in premenopausal women, and high intake of animal protein and red meat was associated with increased risk.

Soy contains several anticarcinogens, but the major influence appears to be its anti-estrogenic effect. Soy products are rich in isoflavones, a phytoestrogen that, when converted by bacteria in the intestine, may suppress estrogen activity. Dietary phytosterol intake differs dramatically among populations. The typical Western diet provides about 80 mg per day, while typical Japanese and vegetarian diets supply up to 400 mg per day.[30] All soy products are not equal with respect to isoflavone content; good choices are tofu, soy milk, tempeh, and soy flours. Soy products, combined with a high-fiber, low-fat diet, may be your best insurance against breast cancer.

Studies on a variety of other foods continue to add to the research. Among the proposed cancer fighters are yogurt, seaweed, garlic, lima beans, green tea, licorice root, flaxseed, parsley, and rosemary.

EXERCISE

The first study specifically designed to investigate whether regular exercise can reduce a woman's risk of breast cancer is being applauded by breast cancer experts. In a group of more than 1,000 women, researchers from the University of Southern California found that women who exercised at least 4 hours a week during their reproductive years had a 58 percent lower breast cancer risk. Those who spent 1 to 3 hours a week exercising cut their risk by 30 percent.[31] Even though the study focused on younger women, who are less likely to develop breast cancer, the results are exciting and hold promise that there are ways women can take health care into their own hands and effect a change.

Previous studies have suggested that physical activity can modify menstrual-cycle patterns and reduce the frequency of ovulation, thus lessening a woman's exposure to estrogen.

POTENTIAL CARCINOGENS

It has been said that the majority of all cancers are caused by the environment and are thus preventable. Cancer has been linked to things we eat, breathe, and are exposed to for a length of time. Without becoming paranoid, it is important that we be aware of potential cancer promoters and avoid them when possible. For example, eating organically grown foods without the addition of synthetic chemicals, pesticides, and herbicides is seriously worth considering.

Potential Sources of Cancer

+ Pesticides (the Environmental Protection Agency identifies 64 pesticides as potentially cancer-causing)

+ Formaldehyde (industrial solvent used in rugs and plastics)

- Coal-tar-based food colorings

- Nitrates and nitrites (found in foods such as hot dogs, bacon, and luncheon meats)

- Smoked foods (bacon, ham, fish, cheese)

- Burned proteins from charred meats

- Cyclamates; saccharin (artificial sweeteners)

- Radiation (low doses accumulate in the body)

- Tobacco (including secondhand smoke)

- Alcohol (taking more than nine drinks per week is associated with increased breast cancer risk)

- Aflatoxins (found in moldy nuts, seeds, and grains)

- DES (diethylstilbestrol, a synthetic estrogen)

- DDT (although banned in the United States, other countries still use this pesticide and send their products to the United States)

Sometimes our fear stops us from doing the very things that could save our lives. Early detection and treatment of breast cancer significantly reduces the probability of death, yet many of us either do not take the time or neglect simple measures. Since 80 percent of breast tumors are discovered by women themselves, practicing breast self-examination can clearly improve a woman's chances for early detection and successful treatment. Monthly breast self-examination is recommended by the National Cancer Institute and the American Cancer Society. In addition, women over the age of 40 should have a mammogram every other year; after 50, they should have yearly mammograms.

11

MORE THAN SKIN DEEP

I have some lines in my face from 50 years of life.
They tell me of years in the sun, of sorrows and joys.
They tell me of time. They tell me I have lived and
that I am still alive. They can't be erased.
They can be softened....
Do I long to be the smooth-skinned, freckle-faced
kid I once was? No. I long for the same thing
today that I longed for then: to be the best
I am able to be.

—KAYLAN PICKFORD, *ALWAYS A WOMAN*

How many of us are willing to admit that we don't always share these lovely sentiments? As mature adults we would like to, but looking into the mirror each morning to find pillow creases etched on our cheeks, we wonder how long it will be until they last all day. What cream can we purchase to smooth out the newly formed lines? What miracle cure will erase these indelible furrows?

The first visible signs of aging appear in the largest and most public organ we have: our skin. A woman may feel young, think young, and act young, but if her face is lined, society will remind her that she has "crossed over" into middle age. And while men seem to profit by their character lines and graying temples, signs of aging are not admired in women.

A woman who is noticeably in the prime of her life may not appear on the cover of national magazines, but in the real world where we all live, I find women are not as obsessed with fine lines and age spots as we are led to believe. We want to look our best, but the panic that fills the literature seems not as pervasive with the majority of women I talk to at seminars. Hopefully, the time will come when we even appreciate the real beauty of the mature look as they do in some foreign countries.

I am not suggesting we give up trying to look as good as we can. How I look has always been important to me and I avail myself of many health and beauty tips. I am saying that we should do all we can to present our best image, then get on with the really important matters of life.

Knowing how our bodies change, and how those changes affect the skin, enables us to take precautions to prevent premature aging and maintain healthy skin.

SKIN CHANGES WITH AGE

How fast the skin ages depends primarily on heredity and partly on a person's lifestyle and skin-care regimen. We can accelerate or postpone signs of aging by manipulating both our external and internal environment. All that we do to and for our bodies is eventually reflected in the skin, which is a mirror of our internal condition. If we choose to live in the fast lane—smoking, drinking to excess, eating junk foods, or worshiping the sun—we will accelerate cellular destruction. If we avoid these excesses, or at least take precautions against their effects, and concentrate on nourishing and rebuilding healthy cells, we can greatly enhance a healthy appearance.

Genetics

Our genetic makeup predetermines much of our aging pattern. People with darker, thicker, more oily skin show fewer wrinkles than people with fair skin, because the heavily pigmented outer layer protects the interior cells from harmful effects of the sun. Men generally do not exhibit fine lines as early as women because their skin is normally thicker and because many of them also follow a skin care program that helps to remove dead skin cells: they shave.

Acne

Most of us consider wrinkles and age spots the major skin problems of the midlife years, but some women experience a return to adolescence in the form of acne. Unsightly pimples sometimes occur in women during perimenopause, when hormones tend to fluctuate most unpredictably. Women who have enjoyed smooth complexions may complain of preteen skin problems. The situation usually takes care of itself in time, but who wants to wait? Some women find that a natural progesterone cream works to combat acne when applied during the second half of their cycles. Severe cases of acne can often be treated with a prescription of retinoic acid (a form of vitamin A). While retinoic acid is effective, it can irritate sensitive skin. Over-the-counter products containing glycolic and citric acids are less expensive and seem to work just as well.

Color Changes

The color of the skin changes with age. Skin pigmentation that was once uniform becomes variegated. Since the skin is susceptible to many influences, it is difficult to determine whether the cause is temporary hormonal imbalance, normal aging, or discoloration due to sun exposure. Age spots—or more appropriately, sun spots, since they are caused by overexposure to the sun—multiply with each passing year. I wish we had all known 30 years ago, when we basked at the beach for hours, that our short-lived tans would come back to haunt us in unsightly patches on our hands and body.

BASIC SKIN ANATOMY

The skin contains one fourth of the body's blood supply, two million or so sweat glands, and even more nerve endings, hair follicles, and sebaceous glands. It performs many necessary functions: helping the body regulate temperature, eliminating waste products and toxins, and protecting the body from invading germs and harmful environmental conditions. It is an organ we must care for both inside and out.

From the moment we are born, the skin is continually renewing itself. At any given time, approximately one fourth of the cells are developing, one half are mature, and one fourth are degenerating. It is said that the human body gets a new outer skin every 27 days from birth to death. That means that what you are doing to or for your body today will show up in your skin next month.

There are three basic layers and several sublayers of skin, and it is deep within the body that healthy skin is conceived. The underskin, filled with blood vessels, nerve endings, fat cells, hair follicles, and connective tissue, is the life-support system that transports nutrients to the visible external layer. Yet our outermost wrapping, or *epidermis*, is often the only part of the skin to which we pay attention.

As we approach menopause, and even sooner for some women, several changes occur in the skin: the underlying fat layer diminishes; collagen and elastin, the skin's structural support system, lose elasticity, gradually yielding less moisture; sweat glands function less vigorously; and the body's natural protection against the sun is reduced. If precautions are not taken internally and externally, a dry, sagging skin is likely to result.

Somewhere around age 35 external evidence of aging shows on the face. Because skin cells are regenerating at a slower rate, as are all body cells, it takes more time for a fresh supply of cells to reach the surface. The dead outer covering that remains is now exposed to the elements for a longer time, resulting in a dehydrated texture. A general loss of oil and moisture make the skin thinner and less flexible. Dryness develops; fine lines and wrinkles emerge.

Many women ask whether estrogen salve or cream will restore their youthful skin. It will to some extent, but only temporarily. Initially, the hormone forces the skin to puff up with water and fat, but over an extended period of time it actually accelerates the breakdown of collagen fibers and blood vessels, thus hastening the loss of skin elasticity. Women using estrogen creams often complain of the same side effects as women who are taking birth-control pills: skin discoloration, rashes, loss of hair, and oily skin. There are far safer ways to bring moisture to your drying cells.

CARING FOR YOUR SKIN FROM WITHIN

The condition of your skin is a fairly accurate gauge of how well you are treating your body. If you have been neglecting your health or have been under greater-than-normal pressure and tension, your skin will let you know. Fortunately, the skin will also respond to positive changes in lifestyle more quickly than any other organ. Learn to deal with your stress; refrain from eating highly processed foods; stop smoking, drinking too much alcohol, and basking in the sun; feed your body with good food and drink plenty of water; and see how your skin reacts.

All vitamins, minerals, and amino acids guard in one way or another against cellular destruction, premature aging, and dry and wrinkled skin.

Nutrients and Skin Health

+ *Vitamin A:* Keeps tissues soft and healthy; guards against scaling and drying; acts as an antioxidant. Vitamins A and D and the mineral zinc may be applied externally for acne-related problems.

+ *B-complex vitamins:* Assist in tissue repair; prevent skin eruptions and hair loss; promote a healthy nervous system; improve circulation; regulate body secretions.

+ *Vitamin B-6:* Aids in the utilization of DNA and RNA (basic to the process of cell reproduction).

+ *Niacin:* Improves circulation and reduces cholesterol; keeps skin, gums, and digestive tissues healthy.

+ *PABA: (para-aminobenzoic acid)* Stimulates intestinal bacteria.

+ *Vitamin C:* Acts as an antioxidant; essential for healing and the formation of collagen; prevents capillary breakage.

+ *Vitamin E:* Acts as an antioxidant; maintains healthy cellular respiration within the muscles.

+ *Essential fatty acids (EFA):* Lubricate skin and hair; prevent dandruff, hair loss, and dry skin.

+ *Iodine:* Essential for normal thyroid activity; necessary for healthy skin, hair, and nails.

+ *Zinc:* Forms collagen for binding cells together as tissues.

+ *Iron:* vital for blood formation; a deficiency can cause dry skin.

A healthy lifestyle is basic to healthy skin. An imbalance or inadequate supply of nutrients can surface on the skin. Chronic dieters who are not eating adequate fat or protein often set themselves up for dry skin and dull hair.

Women who are eating adequately and still notice these conditions need to consider other possibilities. They may have a genetic susceptibility to skin and hair problems. They may have some other medical condition, such as an allergy, that could cause an outward reaction. They may be taking medication that produces changes in the skin or hair as a side effect. Or they may not be absorbing the nutrients their bodies need for a healthy appearance. For example, alcohol hinders the body's ability to absorb several of the B vitamins and disrupts levels of magnesium, potassium, and zinc. Foods high in saturated fats and concentrated sugars demand greater nutrient requirements for absorption. When the diet consists primarily of these types of foods, there is a chance of undernutrition, which can show up on the skin.

KEEPING SKIN HEALTHY
INSIDE AND OUT

Moisture Is Essential

Any element that draws moisture out of the skin, internally or externally, will result in drying and wrinkling. Be aware of aspects of your environment—air conditioning, steam heating, smog, pollution, wind, and sunlight, for example—that affect your skin, and take steps to minimize their dehydrating effects. Avoid using harsh soaps and applying heavy makeup since these, too, reduce natural moisture. As women age they tend to apply extra makeup. Not only is extra makeup not effective for hiding lines and wrinkles, it actually accentuates them. Let the skin breathe by using more moisturizer and less cover-up.

There are many ways to add moisture to your home environment. For instance, you can keep your bathtub filled with water when you are at home; the evaporation of water molecules moistens the air and hydrates the skin. You may want to purchase a large aquarium or fill your home with large plants and bouquets of flowers in oversized vases, enhancing the loveliness of your surroundings while moisturizing your skin.

Skin-Care Products

Adding moisturizer to your skin and protecting the innermost layers becomes more crucial with each passing year. Several safe products on the market can plump up the tissue under the surface of the skin, smooth out lines and wrinkles, and nourish beneath the external layers as well. Which moisturizers will work best for you? It depends on the ingredients and how sensitive your skin is. Don't assume that your moisturizer must be expensive. Consumer Reports tested 48 moisturizers and found that the most effective creams and lotions were the least expensive. Look for the one with the fewest ingredients. The more ingredients in a moisturizer—perfumes, colors, thickeners, emulsifiers—the greater the chance of an allergic reaction.

It was once thought that skin creams did not penetrate the epidermis; now we know this is not true. So before you put anything on your face, check the ingredients to make sure there is nothing harmful in the product, such as alcohol, preservatives, fragrances, coloring, mineral oil, lanolin, and petroleum.

Skin-care product labels are often confusing. Manufacturers are not required to list all ingredients or to indicate whether their sources are natural or synthetic. The use of synthetic ingredients, some of which are proven or suspected carcinogens (quaternium-15, formaldehyde, methylparaben, propylparaben, hexachlorophene, NDELA [nitrosodiethanolamine], TEA [triethanolamine]), is especially problematic in lotions or creams that are designed to stay on the body for long periods of time (12 hours). Immediate allergic reactions and irritations are obvious dangers, but what about the effects of continuous absorption of a potentially harmful chemical over the course of several years?

Certain natural-product manufacturers have recently taken the initiative in developing safe skin-care products. A major improvement is the substitution of natural vegetable oils for mineral oil as the base for body and facial lotions. Mineral oil, a petroleum derivative, is difficult to remove from the skin and can actually clog pores and cause blemishes. As it inhibits the ability of the skin to produce its own oils, it can worsen an already dry skin condition. Olive, wheat germ, safflower, sesame, almond, apricot kernel, and avocado oils are closer in composition to the natural secretions of the skin. Most of them are also rich in linoleic acid, an essential fatty acid that aids in skin-cell renewal. Some manufacturers have also replaced synthetic coloring and scents with herbal extracts and powdered flowers, such as rose, iris, orange blossom, lavender, and camomile.

Exercise

Exercise is vital to vibrant skin and a healthy body. A strenuous workout will increase your circulation, enhance the absorption of nutrients, and stimulate collagen production. According to exercise guru Jane Fonda, "If your budget is limited, you'd do better to invest your money in a regular, sweaty, speed-up-your-heartbeat exercise program than in a lot of expensive hormonal creams, masks, facials, and the like, whose effect will be at best temporary and superficial."[1]

Unconscious Facial Expressions

Many of the facial cracks and creases we develop are due less to aging than to habitual facial expressions and unconscious grimaces. Constant squinting, scowling, smiling, or frowning eventually will leave permanent imprints on the face. To avoid this, some women have even learned to control their smiles. In a television interview, actress Morgan Fairchild demonstrated how she had taught herself to "laugh down" so that crows' feet and other laugh lines would not form on her face. I tried her exercise in front of a mirror and it wasn't easy. On a more practical level, try to avoid unnecessary squinting (especially when outside or reading), and frowning. The furrowed brows and tight lips characteristic of scowlers are among the most unpleasant of all permanent expressions.

Smoking

Over a period of years, lines form around the lips of cigarette smokers because every puff on a cigarette causes the muscles around the mouth to contract. More important, smoking reduces the body's oxygen level, which affects circulation—the primary source of nutrition for all cells. Some authorities suggest that the lower estrogen levels associated with both cigarette smoking and perimenopausal women may further accelerate premature wrinkling. The more heavily you smoke, the more quickly and severely your skin will age. Probably the best all-around good health advice, for a variety of reasons, is to quit smoking.

Alcohol

Alcohol in excess impairs the functioning of the liver, which, in turn, affects every other organ in the body. In the skin, it can contribute to broken or enlarged capillaries near the surface. If you are drinking too much, you will have facial redness or blotchiness, particularly on the cheeks and nose; dullness or poor texture; and excessive wrinkles from the drying effect.

Stress

Stress obviously touches every organ and system in the body, and no skin treatment—aside from massage—will alleviate it. Lack of sleep, overwork, and unresolved issues can manifest on the face and eyes. We have all had times in our lives when no amount of makeup could hide the turbulence. Stress inhibits our digestive processes, prevents absorption of nutrients, and creates a greater need for good nutrition and eating habits. Be kind to your body when it is going through emotional stress, and you will be less likely to see the strain mirrored on your face.

The Sun

Up to 90 percent of the skin changes we once associated with normal aging—including wrinkling, sagging, and a leathery appearance—may actually be a result of damage from the sun and ultraviolet radiation.[2] UV radiation damages the skin's elastic fibers and causes them to thicken while reducing the amount of collagen in the skin, thereby decreasing the skin's ability to hold water. Wrinkling, broken capillaries, age spots, and darker pigmentation may all be more visible with increased exposure to UV radiation.

To protect yourself from premature aging from the sun, avoid direct exposure between the hours of 10:00 A.M. and 3:00 P.M. Wear a hat and long sleeves, and apply a sunscreen anytime you are out for more than a half an hour. You are subject to the sun's rays even when you ride in a car, sit under the shade, or are out on a hazy day.

Sunscreens offer the best protection against both UVA (ultraviolet A) and UVB (ultraviolet B) radiation, but read labels and find one that assures both UVA and UVB or broad-spectrum protection. The shorter UVA rays do the most visible damage, sunburn, and can be more dangerous, causing skin cancer. UVA effects are heightened during the midday hours from May to September. The longer UVB rays are present all day long whenever there is visible light. They may not result in a burn, but when combined with UVA they can also lead to skin cancer.

Experts vary on the best sun protective factor (SPF) rating to use; suggestions range from 15 to 50. If you are fair skinned or have a tendency to burn, a higher number will be more protective.

There is recent debate about whether sunscreen blocks the conversion of vitamin D in the body. This may be of concern if you are cautiously avoiding the sun and fully covering up when you are outside. If no part of your body sees natural light, consider taking a multiple-vitamin supplement with 400 IU of vitamin D.

When you are in the sun, do not use perfume, drink alcohol, or take diuretics, antibiotics, or hormones of any kind. Tetracycline and sulfa drugs produce rashes in the sun; cortisone can cause inflammation around the hair follicles; birth-control pills and hormones can discolor the skin; and Valium can bring on measle-like eruptions if the skin is overexposed. Many other photosensitive drugs and chemicals can cause scales, pimples, or rashes on the skin.

Sun rays are very harmful to the skin and body and can cause skin cancer and melanomas. Heed the warnings and cautiously enjoy your outdoor activities.

A BASIC SKIN-CARE REGIMEN

To learn about treating the aging skin externally, I interviewed Vera Brown, noted beauty and skin-care expert and owner of Vera's Natural Beauty Retreat and Vera's in the Glen in Beverly Glen, California. During our afternoon together, Vera explained the fundamentals that all women should follow to keep their skin healthy, as well as the special problems that arise at menopause.

Not only did Vera teach me the basics of skin care, she offered personal insights into some of the concerns of menopausal women. Many midlife women she sees are extremely unhappy with themselves. They feel their skin and their bodies don't look like they used to, and they feel so bad that it colors their entire life.

Vera gently tells the midlife women who walk through her door that now is the time to start pampering themselves, to give themselves strokes, to be nice to themselves. Instead of looking in the mirror in the morning and being unhappy with what you see, she says, change your outlook. Look at yourself and realize how lucky you are to be alive, how wonderful it is that we now have information about how to feel better and look better, and how blessed we are to live in a time of so many discoveries that will help us through the change. Skin care is vitally important, but don't lose sight of the true meaning of life.

One of the secrets Vera teaches is that skin care isn't just about applying one cream after another. It's about closing the door in the morning and evening to create privacy, to create a time when you will do something only for yourself. Think about your day: you arise, dress, wash your face, eat breakfast, talk on the phone, make appointments, see people—and all your energy is going out, out, out. How often do you sit down, take a deep breath, wash your hands, rub them together, bring the energy back into your face, and do a simple skin-care routine? It may be just washing your face, but use loving strokes, bringing the circulation back into your skin. You will feel better—physically and emotionally—and you will look better. You will be doing something for yourself.

What follows are Vera's own recommendations for a daily skin-care routine.

Cleansing the Skin

Any basic skin-care program starts with a cleanser void of lanolin or mineral oil. You want to use a cleanser that penetrates the skin, because the most important thing about skin care is to keep the skin clean. Nothing is more important. Many women who wear makeup just use soap and water to remove it, and they are not getting a deep enough cleansing. You need a cleanser that actually penetrates the pores. Use a glycerine soap for the face, or another mild soap made without lye, synthetic fragrance, synthetic colors, or preservatives. Fancy soaps are best reserved to impress guests. Cleansing creams also should be free of mineral oil.

Fresheners

After cleansing, use a freshener, void of alcohol, to remove any residue left on the skin. If you don't want to fill your bathroom with skin products, you can apply pure aloe vera or aloe combined with a few drops of lemon juice. There is no need to rinse after the freshener.

Facial Mists

Next, use a facial mist to return moisture to the skin. I use one made up of minerals and rose water, but mineral water will do as well. This step is especially important for dry skin and fine lines. Mineral water reintroduces moisture into the skin, then the cream seeps underneath the skin's surface and pushes out the indentations caused by dehydration. The cream also acts as a seal to keep in moisture. Deep wrinkles you will probably have to live with, unless, of course, you have a face-lift; even then, the surgery is not permanent. You will need another in about five years.

Moisturizers

Apply moisture creams, sparingly, on the dampened face. Use just a little cream, especially at night. So many women going through menopause have extreme sweats; they put lots of cream on at night and all this does is treat their pillowcases. You want your pores to be clean. Let them breathe. You are constantly getting new cells: you slough off the old cells and make new cells. But as one gets older, the cycle slows down. If your cells are clogged, it slows down even more. This is vitally important: when going through menopause, use less cream at night so your pores will stay open. Never go to bed feeling cream on your face. The steps, then, are cleanse, freshen, mist, and moisturize.

Masques

It is very important to slough off the top layer of dead skin so that the new healthy cells can surface. Do this weekly by using facial scrubs, masks, and in extreme conditions, peels. Many products on the market will work, and you can even make ones at home that are equally effective. Here are a couple of my "kitchen facials" from *Vera's Natural Beauty Book*.

Masque for Tightening

1 tablespoon avocado, mashed
2 tablespoons raw honey
2 egg whites

Place ingredients in a blender and process until smooth. Pat onto face. Relax with feet raised while masque acts to tighten skin and increase circulation, about 20 to 30 minutes. Rinse and freshen.

Masques for Dry Skin

Massage some yogurt into clean skin. Add mashed avocado. Leave on the skin for about 20 minutes. Rinse with warm water.

Mash a banana well. Add honey until a creamy consistency is obtained. Apply to a clean face for 20 minutes. Rinse well.

Mash a ripe papaya. Add the white of an egg, and mix until creamy. Apply to the face for 20 minutes. Rinse well.

CARING FOR THE REST OF YOUR BODY

So far, we have focused on facial skin, but we should not neglect the rest of the body. When it comes to total body relaxation, nothing compares to a long, hot soak in the tub. Baths can be relaxing and invigorating for the mind as well as the body. Some experts claim that baths are too drying for the skin, but they need not be if you moisturize afterward.

To make your bath special, add natural ingredients to the water for various effects. Cleopatra used milk in her bath; you might want to try adding a quart of milk to your bath water. For very dry skin, try one-half cup of sesame oil. Some women like the fragrance and feeling that freshly brewed herbs offer. Brew your favorite combination (try rosemary, thyme, and lavender flowers) in a bowl, steep for about 20 minutes, strain, and add the liquid to your bath. If you are in the mood for an invigorating bath, if your muscles are aching from aerobics, or if you are tired or have a sunburn, try one cup of natural apple cider vinegar in your water. To really energize your body as well as your spirits, shower after soaking, alternating hot and cold sprays.

After soaking, use a loofah sponge to remove the dry, dead cells from the outer layer of skin. The scrub will invigorate you, as it increases blood circulation and tones the skin.

HAIR CARE

Hair is an extension of the skin, and it responds to changing hormones and normal aging in characteristic ways. Like the skin, hair reflects your state of health. Philip Kingsley, a British specialist in scalp and hair science, writes, "If you're not eating properly, or exercising regularly, or if you've been under a great deal of stress, the effects are bound to show up on your hair."[3]

Hair follicles are nourished deep beneath the surface of the skin, so if you have problems with dull, dry, or limp hair, check your diet and daily habits before spending your entire paycheck on external conditioners and treatments. External treatments may enhance the hair's manageability and work with the nutritional treatments recommended here—and they need not always be expensive.

Hormonal Changes and Hair Growth

At menopause, some women experience hair loss from their heads and pubic area while others find new growth in places they have never seen it before: their chin, upper lip, chest, and abdomen. While facial hair may be unsightly and embarrassing, it is not a sign of emerging masculine tendencies. It indicates only a reversal in the ratio of female to male hormones, both of which we all— men and women—share. Since estrogen is not dominant following menopause, hair follicles tend to follow a male growth-distribution pattern.

Logical reasoning would suggest that taking more estrogen would reestablish the ratio of hormones and therefore the hair growth pattern. Unfortunately, estrogen does not reverse the process, but it may prevent further hair growth. Progesterone cream also seems to be of some benefit in slowing down the growth of facial and body hair, but it takes time, up to six months. The best alternative may be topical: to bleach the hair if it is dark, or remove it through shaving, waxing, depilatories, or electrolysis.

Nutritional Factors Related to Problem Hair

Sudden hair loss, or hair that is dry, greasy, or lusterless, may not always be hormonally related; it may be nutritionally induced. Healthy hair depends on a delicate balance of protein within the hair shaft and oil outside the hair shaft. If the follicles are inadequately nourished, any number of symptoms might emerge. For example, if your hair feels unusually greasy, it may indicate a diet too rich in animal fat. Eliminating red meat, butter, fried foods, and pastries from your diet may be all that is necessary to reestablish chemical equilibrium. Dry hair frequently responds to foods rich in B vitamins, vitamin E, vitamin A, and a daily dose (2 teaspoons) of vegetable oil. Hair loss may be checked by adding high-quality protein to and eliminating junk foods from your diet, and supplementing with iron and zinc.

Fasting and fad dieting over the years often lead to hair thinning and loss. Past years of depletion can intensify a woman's present needs for nutrients; she will need greater amounts of all vitamins and minerals than if she had been adequately nourished all along.

It is easy to overlook certain nutrients in your diet. For example, a subtle complication of the vegetarian diet, especially one that does not include egg and milk products, is the lack of the amino acid methionine.[4] Even a slight deficiency in this nutrient over a period of time may result in loss of hair.

Certain drugs, most notably birth-control pills, have been implicated in hair loss. If you are taking hormonal drugs, it would be wise to increase your intake of foods containing sulfur, the B-complex vitamins, and zinc.

Essential fatty acids are especially important to menopausal women since they provide moisture to all tissues of the body as well as to the skin and hair. Incorporate more whole, raw seeds and nuts in your diet; eat fresh fish several times a week; and for supplementation add 1 to 2 teaspoons of flaxseed oil to salads or vegetables. Flaxseed oil also comes in capsules; 2 to 8 a day will replace moisture in your skin and hair and may make an appreciable difference in the way you look and feel.

Stress endured over a long period of time or a sudden traumatic experience may cause sudden hair loss or scalp disorders. However, the hair will usually return to normal when the situation has subsided. You can aid the process by making your diet rich in B-complex vitamins, vitamins E and C, and folic acid.

The Bottom Line for Healthy Skin and Hair

+ Keep out of the direct sun, and protect your skin with hats and sunscreen.

+ Don't smoke.

+ Minimize chemical drinks (coffee, tea, cola, diet drinks, and alcohol).

+ Drink plenty of water—at least 2 quarts per day.

+ Don't lose weight too rapidly (2 pounds a week at the most).

+ Eat high-quality protein and complex carbohydrates.

+ Minimize your intake of excess oil, saturated fats, and hydrogenated spreads.

+ Reduce sugar and refined and enriched flours and grains in your diet.

+ Keep the air in your home moist (especially if you live in a dry climate, work in an air-conditioned building, or fly often). Spray mists of water to help bring moisture back to your face.

+ Supplement your diet, emphasizing antioxidants (vitamins A, C, and E, and the mineral selenium) and essential oils like flaxseed oil.

+ Exercise regularly.

12

WEIGHT CONTROL

The sad thing is that too many people
ignore the basics in the search
for the esoteric.
—COVERT BAILEY

If we are not careful, middle-age spread can creep up on any of us. After 30, the body starts to change metabolically; muscle tissue decreases, and the body's basal metabolic rate (BMR), the rate at which we burn calories, slows down. By some estimates, the BMR decreases about 2 percent each decade, which means by age 80, we need to take in 200 fewer calories each day (see Figure 5). For most women this will not be enough of a reduction. Because their activity level has also lessened, maintaining the same weight requires further reduction in food intake. There is no way around it: to maintain our weight, we must alter our eating habits and remain physically active.

Obviously, monitoring your weight throughout your life is better than discovering at menopause that you have a serious problem. Menopause brings enough issues to contend with; you don't need to compound the situation by having to diet as well. Sometimes, I think the best way to maintain your figure is to vow never to buy a larger size in clothes. You may not be eating more than you normally do, but your body will tell you the time has come to make adjustments.

A bathroom scale is not an accurate indicator of fitness or optimum weight. In fact, I suggest you throw out your scale. It does

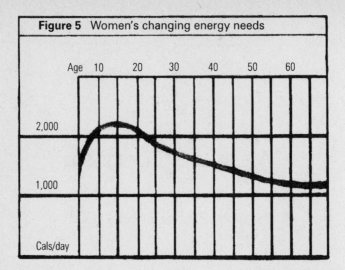

Figure 5 Women's changing energy needs

not tell you how your body should look or how healthy you are. Worst of all, it can become a constant source of anxiety and guilt.

How important is keeping our weight down after 50? Certainly, a few additional pounds won't harm most women, but I think the operative word here is *few*. Studies show that the pounds you put on in midlife may be more harmful than any extra weight you carried in your early adult years. Women who gain weight later in life are at a higher risk for heart disease than those who have carried the weight all their lives. Being overweight to the point of obesity is extremely high risk, and is associated with heart disease, high blood pressure, adult-onset diabetes, and certain types of cancer (notably breast, endometrial, and colon cancers).

National surveys indicate that the trend for American adults in the last decade is toward being overweight.[1] Why is this, given the explosion of weight-loss programs, diet drinks, low-fat foods, and exercise clubs? The basic reason is simple: diets that are very different from your natural way of eating do not work.

Why Americans are Overweight and Overfat

+ Unhealthy eating habits (eating high-fat foods, overeating, and skipping meals) can promote weight gain and prevent weight loss.

✦ Most people miscalculate what they eat by 18 percent.

✦ The more you diet and regain weight, the harder it is to lose weight subsequently. Your metabolic rate may decrease by as much as 15 to 20 percent after only a 6-percent decrease in weight, so it becomes harder for you to burn off calories the next time around.

✦ There may be a link between yo-yo dieting and choosing a high-fat diet.

✦ A survey of the recreational habits of Americans found that the first 13 most popular activities—among them, watching TV or videos and reading books—are inactive. The fourteenth is walking.

✦ It is harder for women to lose weight and easier for them to gain weight than it is for men. Estrogen is pro-fat: the more fat you store, the more estrogen you make; the more estrogen you make, the more fat you store.

This past decade I worked for two major diet enterprises, one a medically supervised fasting program and the other a popular food-control weight-loss center. People did lose weight in record amounts, and I felt gratified that I had been helpful in their efforts. When they regained their weight—often with several additional pounds—the excitement subsided. From this experience, and my studies of the literature for answers, I think I have found some reasons why people cannot maintain weight loss.

MOST DIETS DON'T WORK

Anyone who has agonized over successive diets knows they do not help keep the weight off permanently. You lose pounds, but the loss is temporary; once you resume your normal eating habits the fat finds its way back.

There are two primary reasons diets fail. First, most diets are foreign to the way people normally eat. Many dieters carefully follow strict low-calorie menus or concoct special drinks until the scale shows the right numbers, then they go back to potato chips, croissants, and hot-fudge sundaes because they cannot maintain the unnatural rigidness of the diet. A diet must change your *approach* to eating in the long term, or you will not maintain weight loss.

Second, very low caloric intake changes the body metabolism in a way that promotes weight gain. When you go on a crash diet of, say, nothing but grapefruit and hard-boiled eggs, you actually encourage the storage of fat. As caloric intake is drastically reduced, the body does everything it can to conserve energy. It lowers the metabolic rate to protect you from starving. The more quickly pounds dissolve (especially if it is more than two pounds a week), the more intensely the body hoards its fat. You may lose weight initially, but the pounds you are burning are from your lean muscle tissue rather than from fat stores. Biochemically, your body changes. When muscle mass is decreased, the basal metabolic rate slows down. This means you are burning fewer calories than you did before you started dieting. So, when you return to "normal" eating, it is even easier to gain weight than it was before.

Crash diets are counterproductive in more ways than one. Reducing calories to bare-minimum levels usually means reducing nutrient stores as well. When the system is depleted of its vitamins and minerals, it triggers the appetite mechanism in the brain to replenish its supply. Result? You are starved, so you eat. Bingeing and compulsive eating are common among professional dieters.

When women "blitz," they often cut fat out of their plans entirely. This, too, is both unhealthy and ineffective. A good rule is never to follow any diet that eliminates an entire food group— fats, carbohydrates, or proteins. If you eliminate fats completely, you may develop dry and brittle hair, dandruff, swelling in the hands and feet, acne, and loss of sex drive. Ironically, one essential fatty acid, linoleic acid, helps burn fat. Restrict your intake of fats—but do not eliminate them entirely.

Frequent and drastic dieting is an emotional nightmare for many women. The Mayo Clinic studied a group of young, healthy women, women who had no reason to lose weight but who volunteered for the sake of research. They lived together in the clinic, ate a restricted diet, and were tested continually for side effects. "Before three months had passed, the women's personalities underwent startling changes. They began to quarrel endlessly with one another, experienced unprovoked feelings of anxiety, persecution, and hostility. Some suffered nightmares; others felt extreme panic at times . . . . Their memories became faulty; they were clumsy and had trouble paying attention to assigned tasks."[2] Remember, before the experiment these women were emotionally healthy and not overweight; they were exposed to only one reducing diet, yet they suffered great anxiety. (Other factors, such as living in the clinic with the group tested, could also have contributed to these changes.)

Repeated dieting can be dangerous. Analyzing 32 years of data from the Framingham Heart Study in Massachusetts, researchers looked at weight changes in more than 3,000 men and women. They found that people whose weight fluctuated often or dramatically doubled their risk for developing heart disease and increased their rate of premature death.[3] Equally startling was the finding that relatively thin people were as much at risk as the overweight. This study does not suggest that weight loss is harmful, but that it should be taken seriously.

Dieting is a stress on the body, both physically and emotionally. Individuals who experiment with one diet after another are forced to deal not only with the normal anxiety of dieting but with the psychological repercussions of failing, the feelings of guilt, frustration, and ego deflation. Crash diets, fad diets, and minimum-calorie diets are unhealthful for the mind as well as for the body. Their benefits are temporary at best; their side effects are multiple and potentially dangerous. So what's the solution?

THE PROPER ATTITUDE

The place to begin is with one's basic attitude toward dieting and good health. We live in a society in which we are conditioned to expect instant results. Over-the-counter remedies are available for almost every ache and pain. For a headache, an upset stomach, or a runny nose, we simply take a pill. If we are overweight, our response is no different. Where's that magic solution—the pill that promises to dissolve our unwanted bulges while we sleep? Clearly, the dollars we shell out for such overnight cures would be far better spent on whole, nutritious foods and a pair of walking shoes.

You cannot keep pounds off your body permanently until you realize that the foods you eat on your "weight-loss program" must be similar to the foods you will choose for the rest of your life. A diet is not temporary; it is a way of living that you maintain on a regular basis. The emphasis needs to be changed from short-term deprivation to long-term change.

It is necessary to retrain your mind to focus on "eating for life" those foods that cause you to feel good, alive, energetic, young, and positive about yourself. It is an attitude of "what is good for my wonderful body" rather than "what do I have to give up so I can lose 10 pounds by Saturday night."

All eating behaviors are learned, and can be unlearned. Therefore, unhealthy eating habits can be replaced with more constructive patterns. This sounds easier than it is, however. Destructive thoughts and practices concerning food and eating have become so much a part of our lives that we don't even realize they exist. Before making changes, we need to take some time, make a personal inventory, and evaluate our attitudes and behaviors about food. We need to examine why we eat or overeat, when we eat, and what we may be doing in terms of our eating that may be preventing us from losing weight.

I discussed the reasons for failed diets with psychologist and weight-loss expert, Bobbe Sommer, and it is her belief that our present-day thought patterns concerning food originate in early childhood. Dr. Sommer suggested that much of what we believe to be true may be, in actuality, lies. For example, when we were young and experienced actual hunger, we knew crying would get us prompt attention. Someone would soon come along and shove a warm bottle in our mouth, and we were soon sated. At the same time we were also cuddled and held close. Now examine this association between food, security, and love only 40 years later. We may still be responding to this associative conditioning. Sometimes when we think we are hungry, we are really experiencing another emotion that is triggering feelings of uneasiness in our abdominal area. We reach for our famous tension reducer, because it worked so well 40 years ago. We have misconstrued the feelings of anxiety in the "pit of our stomach" to be hunger pangs and have acted inappropriately.

Dr. Sommer's theory is that "being fat may be the result of faulty problem solving, at least in some people." Many people attempt to solve their current problems with methods that were appropriate once but no longer serve them well—and they will remain caught in this syndrome until they identify their true emotions. Once they bring the hidden feelings to the level of awareness, they can take action. By unraveling childhood emotions and associations they can be free of the old compulsion to eat whenever they feel a pang in the tummy.

For some people, accepting that their weight problem may lie within the subconscious is frightening. But if this is a primary source of the problem, other programs probably will not work. Not everyone requires extensive therapy, but some people will greatly benefit. For the majority, just raising their own awareness of when they eat or overeat is enough. There are place cues (movies = buttered popcorn and candy), activity cues (watching television = leftovers and cake), and time cues (the hour before dinner = munchies and glasses of wine). Overweight people are much more susceptible to external or environmental cues. Dr. Sommer strongly recommends a daily journal as a tool for bringing one's feelings to the surface and ultimately taking control of behaviors that interfere with our lives.

There are some universal attitudes or childhood messages concerning food that unconsciously destroy our best intentions.

+ I must eat everything on my plate. (*What if you're full?*)

+ It's wasteful to throw food away. (*What if you really don't like it?*)

+ I can't imagine myself thin. (*Keep practicing.*)

+ I'm just a fast eater. (*You will enjoy your food longer if you savor each bite.*)

+ I won't enjoy eating if I have to change. (*Try it first and see.*)

+ I've never kept my weight off. I was meant to be fat. (*There are reasons the weight has returned after dieting. Find out what they are.*)

All of these messages defeat permanent weight loss. If you believe any of them, at all, you need to substitute new, more positive thought patterns.

EVALUATING YOUR EATING HABITS

People eat for countless reasons that have nothing to do with hunger. We eat to be sociable, to be accepted. We eat out of boredom, frustration, anger, a need for acceptance, and habit—most of all habit. And often we are not even conscious of what we are doing. How many cups of coffee and halves of doughnuts did you devour when you were pouring out your soul to your neighbor? As you wait for dinner to be served, do you keep track of the rolls and butter you accept or the glasses of wine poured for you?

Research has shown that many overweight women have completely lost the sensation of hunger: they cannot differentiate it from other feelings. Eating has become their universal response to all stimulation. Therefore, no matter what or how they feel, they seek to satisfy themselves with food. One of the first aspects of food control is to determine when you are eating out of genuine hunger and when you are eating to fulfill a secondary need.

I find charting eating habits to be the best way to record caloric intake as well as to track faulty eating patterns. I sense your reluctance at the mere thought of all that work, and I hear your response: I know what I eat and I don't have the time. Well, several studies have proven you wrong. Diet histories show that women underestimate their daily intake by 500 to 900 calories. When I am struggling with zippers and wondering why, I go back to charting, and find the dietary culprits in no time.

To use the charting method, write down—and be specific—everything you eat and drink for three weeks. (See the sample chart on page 203.) This time frame is necessary to cover a variety of occasions and experiences—your period, social situations, family get-togethers—that can affect your eating habits. You will be amazed at the different kinds of foods you select when you are alone or with relatives, at parties, and during your period. Most people eat about 15 foods regularly, so the task won't take that long. It is not what you eat occasionally that adds up; it is what you do on a daily basis.

DAILY EATING BEHAVIOR DIARY

Time	Food (type and quantity)	Activity while eating	Location	Thoughts and feelings	Action plan
6:00 AM	juice	getting dressed	bedroom	no time to eat	wake up 15 minutes earlier tomorrow
10:00 AM	2 doughnuts; coffee	talking to coworker	lunchroom	low energy; needed a pickup; ate too fast	(1) eat one doughnut more slowly (2) get muffin or bring bagel
1:00 PM	tostada with sour cream and guacamole; cola; cheesecake	read news-paper and ate alone	restaurant	eat something healthful; need dessert	(1) take sour cream off food and just taste guacamole (2) don't eat shell (3) take mints to satisfy sweet tooth
3:00 PM	diet soda	working	work	thirsty; just want something	water is a better choice
8:00 PM	3–4 glasses white wine; chips; vegetables and dip; salad with dressing; 2 rolls with butter; chicken in cream sauce; steamed vegetables; rice; chocolate cake; coffee with cream	dinner meeting	hotel banquet room	these people make me nervous; look busy, eat; I paid for this food so I'm going to eat it	(1) wine spritzer (2) sip wine more slowly (3) eat vegetables without dip (4) just taste roll and butter (5) scrape most of cream sauce off food (6) just taste cake (7) take coffee black

For a *free* blank chart that you can copy, write or call the publisher. See last page for details.

In addition to the *kinds* and *amounts* of food you eat, record the *time* that you ate and *what* you were doing (watching TV, reading the paper, getting dressed, feeding the baby). Often, when we are involved in another activity, we forget that we have eaten, and repeat the process shortly thereafter. Finally, record how you *felt* while you were eating: relaxed, bored, angry, upset, nervous, or nothing in particular? Were you really hungry, or did you have some other need to meet?

By the time you complete the three weeks, you will know a great deal more about your day-to-day eating patterns. How much of your diet is nutrient-rich foods and how much is junk food? You will have a greater appreciation of the nutrient density of your diet, how many fruits and vegetables you eat, and the amount of fiber you get in a day or week. It is an exercise that is well worth your time.

Just as important as what, where, and why you eat is how often you eat. Do you go all day without eating and then gorge before going to bed? Barbara Edelstein, author of *The Woman Doctor's Medical Guide*, believes strongly in eating balanced meals throughout the day. In her opinion, the female body cannot metabolize more than a certain number of calories per meal; if this amount is exceeded the excess will be stored as fat.[4] While the idea of eating several meals may sound counterproductive to losing weight, it really is not. The following study cited by Dr. Edelstein illustrates this important concept.

Volunteers were divided into four groups and given a basic calorie-restricted diet. The first group balanced 1,000 calories among three meals throughout the day and lost two pounds per week. The second group ate no breakfast, had 250 calories for lunch, and 500 calories for dinner. They, too, lost two pounds, though they consumed only 750 calories. The third group ate only 500 calories—all for dinner—and lost the same amount. Personally, I would rather have the freedom to eat twice as much if the weight loss is the same. The fourth group consumed 1,000 calories, all at dinner, and lost less weight than the other groups. So it does appear that small but frequent meals spread throughout the day are more conducive to weight loss and health.

If you have a weight challenge it is vital to examine the whats, whens, and whys of your eating behavior. Until you know, you cannot make informed choices and changes. Once you have determined what you are eating or doing that promotes weight gain, you can develop a plan for change. Start by considering foods on your chart that do not add either nutritional or emotional value to your eating pleasure. Are there any you can totally eliminate? What about placing some in a special-occasion category? Don't choose something you can't go one day without. Make it easy for yourself. For example, forego that fifth cookie, or pre-dinner wine and munchies. Another way of cutting down calories and fat is to substitute lower-calorie foods for things you regularly eat. Sometimes this works and sometimes it doesn't. If the taste and sensual pleasure are missing from a substitution, pass it up. Don't force yourself to eat foods you don't like; it won't work.

Too many of us have tried to lose weight through stringent dieting or unrealistic exercise programs. When goals are not met, discouragement and depression follow. Changing our mindset to realistic lifestyle changes may not come naturally, as we have grown up thinking that we must starve or eat strange things to lose weight. But I have seen how small, seemingly insignificant modifications in food patterns, combined with moderate physical activity, can alter a woman's life dramatically. Not only do they feel better physically, but the fact they did it themselves boosts their self-image. You really can do it yourself—with little time and effort.

It is important to start slowly—just the opposite of commercial programs, which promise instant results. Actually, the faster you lose, the faster you regain. Get used to the idea that you are making *permanent* changes, by charting and thinking about what might realistically work for you. Changing habits permanently is never easy; consider one modification at a time, and when you feel comfortable with one success, move on to the next goal.

WHERE'S THE FAT HIDING?

All recent studies arrive at this central conclusion: fat is the key to both weight loss and weight gain. Since fat contains more calories per gram than either protein or carbohydrates, when you forego fat, you substantially cut down on calories.

Calories in Foods

FOOD	CALORIES/GRAM
Protein	4
Carbohydrates	4
Fat	9

Fat further encourages fatness by its metabolic effect. While it takes 25 percent of the energy in protein and carbohydrates to transform them into substances the body uses, a similar conversion only takes 3 percent of the energy in fat. This means that 97 percent of fat calories can be stored immediately. "A minute on the lips, forever on the hips" is oh, so true for fat.

An average woman consumes 80 to 100 grams fat per day. Optimal for good health as well as weight loss is between 25 to 50 grams per day. If you want a more specific number, you can calculate your optimal daily fat intake from the total number of calories you ingest in a day. Multiply your total daily caloric intake by the optimal percentage of fat calories (20–25 percent) and divide the result by 9 (the calories in 1 gram of fat). (See page 168 for an example.)

Fat intake is relatively easy to monitor given the number of books on the market listing fat grams for every kind of food. More detailed food labels have greatly enhanced our awareness. But you will need those three-week food records first. You don't have to continue them for the rest of your life, only until you get a feeling for what you are eating and those areas that need revamping.

You will find that when you start eating lower-fat foods, you can increase your quantities and still not gain weight. To give you some appreciation for the amounts of food you can eat that may equal a high-fat food, look at the following list. I love to demonstrate this with plates of all these items, but I think you will get the idea.

Lowering fat in your diet does not have to alter your lifestyle appreciably and may not be as difficult as you imagine. A two-year feasibility study was conducted to see whether a group of women aged 45 to 69 could practically reduce the fat content of their diet from the typical 39 percent to 20 percent using regular, readily available food (no specific diet foods). Not only did they lose the weight, but they maintained it after a two-year follow-up term.[5] The researchers concluded that fat-controlled diets are effective and practical, since American women can use foods that are easily at hand.

MINOR LIFESTYLE CHANGES
MAKE MAJOR DIFFERENCES

Cutting down on fat will allow you to lose weight—not in record time, but that's not the point. The goal is to take it off slowly and then maintain. If you eliminate 1 tablespoon of butter a day, an amount that easily covers two slices of toast, in one year you would lose 10 pounds. Consider the following chart as you think about what to cut out of your diet to produce lasting results

EXERCISE IS A MUST

Exercise is a major factor for long-term weight loss.[6] Studies confirm that maintaining a regular exercise program is the surest way of determining future success. Cutting calories and fat without adding exercise may cause you to lose as much lean muscle tissue as you do fat. A person who drops 20 pounds from dieting alone will often lose as much as 10 pounds of muscle. While this looks good on the scales, the muscle loss lowers metabolic rate and thus increases the chances of regaining the weight.

Exercise builds muscle mass, thereby raising the BMR. Even moderate exercise increases the metabolic rate three to eight times. And there is a residual effect of regular exercise that keeps the metabolic rate higher than normal for several hours afterward, allowing you to burn more calories even when you are not working at it.

Exercise can change the body's chemistry. When biopsies from endurance athletes were compared to those of un-

What Could You Eat if You Gave up a Bacon Cheeseburger?

FOOD	FAT GRAMS
Bacon cheeseburger	63
Charbroiled chicken sandwich	7
Bagel	12
Potato	0
Apple	0
Banana	0
1 cup spaghetti	1
1/2 cup marinara sauce	4
Chicken leg	9
Turkey sandwich (no mayo)	7
1 slice pizza (small)	5
Corn tortilla	1
Flour tortilla	3
1 oz. cheese	9
1 egg	7
1/2 cup cereal	2
3 pancakes (small)	2
2 low-fat cupcakes	4
Total	**63**

Reduce Amounts of High-Fat Foods

FOOD	CALORIES	FAT GRAMS
butter (1 Tbsp.)	100	12
cheese (1 oz.)	100	9
mayonnaise (1 Tbsp.)	100	11
potato chips (1 oz.)	150	11
nuts (1 cup)	850	80
Hershey's chocolate (2.6 oz)	390	20

Replace with Lower-Calorie, Lower-Fat Foods

TRY	INSTEAD OF
1 slice whole-wheat toast (71 calories/ 1 fat gram)	1 croissant (300 calories/ 12 fat grams)
4 cups of popcorn (109/0)	potato chips (300/22)
7 oz. broiled fish (175/2)	7 oz. fried fish (525/18)
1/2 cup Dreyer's Lite (100/4)	1/2 cup Häagen-Daz (270/17)
1 corn tortilla (50/1)	1 flour tortilla (150/4)
2 Tbsp. broth (0/0)	2 Tbsp. cooking oil (240/27)
3 oz. turkey sausage (150/0)	3 oz. pork sausage (300/25)
3 oz. skinless baked chicken (160/4)	3 oz. fried chicken (230/14)

trained college students, it was found that the athletes had a greater number of fat-burning enzymes. After the untrained person engaged in endurance exercise for several months, their enzymes increased too. Apparently, in people who exercise regularly, the body "revs up" the metabolic system to burn fat more efficiently while protecting the muscle tissue.

Exercise affects many hormonal systems in the body. It increases the responsiveness of cells to insulin so that the insulin does not cause increased fat storage. Stress-related hormones like adrenalin and cortisol are metabolized by exercise, which decreases their effect on fat storage. Endorphins secreted in the brain as a result of endurance exercise create a feeling of well-being, and alleviate depression. Many chemical reactions occur from continued exercise that change the body from one that likes to store fat to one that likes to burn fat.

There is no alternative to a sound exercise program for burning fat. It must be included in any weight-loss program.

A FEW MORE TIPS

A few other tips may be helpful as you plan your weight-loss strategy. No advice is universal, so take what works for you and throw out the rest.

Creating New Eating Habits

◆ Eat at least three meals a day. Skipping meals promotes the starvation response and the storage of fat.

◆ Get into the habit of talking to your food. Before eating, ask, "Do I want you? Do I need you? Are you going to make me feel good or bad when I'm finished?"

◆ Eat without distractions: no TV, radio, newspaper, or book. Concentrate on the food.

◆ Create a relaxing, positive environment.

◆ Eat slowly, enjoying the aroma, color, taste, and texture of the food.

◆ Eat sitting down. You will be less likely to forget what has gone into your mouth.

◆ Practice leaving a few bites on your plate at each meal. This teaches self-control.

◆ Eat with friends, family, or coworkers. Overweight people often feel they must prove to others they are trying to lose weight, so they limit their selections to lettuce and cottage cheese in public, only to binge in solitude. Eat your favorite foods with your friends. Chances are you won't feel the need to overeat later.

◆ Make a list of activities that make you feel good: reading a novel; going to a concert, play, or movie; calling a friend; watching soap operas; getting a facial or massage; going shopping.

◆ If you *must* have a hot-fudge sundae, go ahead. But don't chastise yourself. There's no place for guilt in weight management.

◆ Start a support group or find a friend who will walk with you and listen to your struggles. Social support has been associated with success in weight loss.

13

Exercise for Life

I don't bust my buns working out
every day for nothing.

—CHER

Exercise is as important to a healthy body as good food.
Preventing menopausal symptoms and dealing with the
associated problems of aging involves more than what we
do or don't eat. To be well prepared for midlife we must engage in
some form of physical exercise. "Virtually all the evidence we have
points in the same direction," says Jack Wilmore, director of the
Exercise and Sport Sciences Laboratory, University of Arizona.
"Exercise makes you healthier and may impact longevity. It's time
to become more aggressive in using exercise to improve overall
health."[1]

Exercise literally can save your life; without it, your body
deteriorates. If you are inactive during your adult years, your bones
will decalcify, leading to osteoporosis. Taking time out of your day
to attend an exercise class, take a walk, or jog is not frivolous; it is
essential.

If you want strong bones to support your frame and firm
muscles to protect your internal organs when you reach 50, you
should start your program early. But it is never too late to benefit
from exercise; quite the contrary, with conditioning, you can have
stronger muscles at 50 than you did at 30. I do, and Jane Fonda says
her body was in better shape at 49 than at 20. But optimum results
come from planned preparation, not last-minute desperation.

Most people are aware of the role exercise plays in weight loss. We are also familiar with its influence on the muscle-bone system. But there is more—much more—that exercise can do for your body, mind, and spirit. When you are working the entire body, the effects radiate throughout each and every organ, tissue, and cell.

Benefits of Sustained, Regular Exercise

+ When you exercise vigorously you bring oxygen to every cell of the body, improving circulation, reducing fatigue, creating energy, and increasing your capacity for handling stress.

+ Harvard studies show that aerobic exercise is a practical way to treat the emotional stress of daily living. It can reduce depression and give you a feeling of well-being.

+ Regular exercise can prolong life, according to Ralph Passenbarger, Jr., of the Stanford University School of Medicine: "For each hour of physical activity, you can expect to live that hour over—and live one or two more hours to boot."[2]

+ Physical activity stimulates digestion and increases the absorption of nutrients. A study performed by Gail Butterfield of the University of Southern California showed that active women had appreciably more vitamin C and iron in their bloodstream than did sedentary women.[3]

+ Exercise guards against constipation.

+ Exercise helps you to sleep soundly.

+ For women, exercise can help bring the hormones to a normal level, greatly reducing menstrual cramps, PMS, and hot flashes.

+ Exercise helps the adrenal glands to convert androstenadione into estrone, the major source of estrogen after menopause, allowing for a smoother transition.

+ Exercise is vital to weight control: it diminishes appetite, burns calories, builds muscle, and speeds up body metabolism.

+ Aerobic exercise stimulates new bone formation, thus warding off osteoporosis.

+ Exercise greatly reduces the risk of heart disease. Researchers at the University of North Carolina have found that inactive women are three times more likely to die prematurely from heart disease than the physically active.[4]

+ Exercise lowers the incidence of cancer. In a landmark study at Harvard University, female athletes were found to have 50 percent less incidence of breast cancer and 60 percent less cancer of the uterus, ovaries, cervix, and vagina than nonathletes.

+ Exercise reduces the risk of adult-onset diabetes by improving one's ability to utilize sugar in the blood.

+ Exercise helps prevent joint stiffness, arthritis, and lower-back pain.

Exercise comes in many forms. The kind that's best for you depends on your age, level of fitness, and interests. Evaluate your goals before you buy shoes or equipment or join a health club. Make sure that what you choose is something you want to pursue and can easily incorporate into your life. Your exercise program should not be approached like a fad diet—a temporary inconvenience you tolerate until you reach a desired goal. It should be something you can enjoy. To derive permanent benefits, you need to continue a regular program for the rest of your life. The kind of exercise you choose today may change as you expand your goals and improve your level of fitness, and you should keep adjusting your routines to accommodate your changing needs.

Women approaching menopause have specific fitness needs that can best be met by three basic forms of exercise: aerobic conditioning, muscle strengthening, and stretching. Within these groups, however, are endless variations; you can choose the ones you like and that best fit your schedule.

AEROBIC EXERCISE

The great thing about aerobic activity is that it can be completely individual, matched to your state of health. You do not have to join an arduous dance class or run 10 miles to get into shape. If you are middle-aged, or even a young but unfit woman, simply walking briskly will elevate your heart rate and give you the training effect you require.

Aerobic exercise involves the large muscles of the body and raises the breathing and heart rates, which have a systemic effect throughout the body. Jogging or fast walking works not only the leg muscles, but touches your heart, lungs, bones, and all other organs as well.

For weight control, exercising aerobically must be the number one priority. Even though an aerobic exercise burns little fat during the exercise itself, it has tremendous effects on the metabolization of fat, including fat storage and the ability of muscles to burn fat. You may successfully lose pounds for a while on a low-calorie diet, but it will eventually cease to work because of lost muscle tissue and the need to cut calorie consumption to an unhealthy level for continued loss.

Aerobic means "depending on oxygen." It is used by fitness specialists to describe exercises that increase breathing and pulse rates and produce predictable changes in the body (such as burning calories, strengthening the cardiovascular system, and toning the muscles). All aerobic exercises have one thing in common: as your muscles work hard, they demand and use more oxygen. The main objective of an aerobic exercise program, according to "the father of aerobics," Kenneth Cooper, is to increase the amount of oxygen the body can process within a given time. Dr. Cooper calls this maximum amount *aerobic capacity*. It is dependent upon the ability to (1) rapidly breathe large amounts of air, (2) forcefully deliver large volumes of blood, and (3) effectively deliver oxygen to all parts of the body. Because it reflects the condition of the vital organs, aerobic capacity is often considered the best index of overall physical fitness.[5]

For your exercise workout to be aerobic, you must (1) engage in continuous activity (not stop-and-start) that works the muscles and the heart for a period of 15 to 30 minutes; (2) exercise at a specified intensity; and (3) practice the exercise regularly—at least three times a week to maintain, five times to improve.

How hard you exercise is a personal decision that should be based on your heart rate. As intensity increases, oxygen demand goes up and your heart beats faster. The point is to keep within a specified range (your *training rate*) during the conditioning period.

It is important to determine the training rate that is right for you. You can do this by taking your pulse during the aerobic workout. If the exercise has truly been aerobic, your pulse will register between 60 and 80 percent of your maximum heart rate (MHR), which is around 220 beats a minute less your age. The formula used to determine the training rate is based on your MHR and the percentage increase you want to achieve. The following example is for a person 45 years old:

$$220-45 \ \ = 175 \ (\text{maximum heart rate})$$

$$175 \times .60 = 105 \ \text{beats per minute}$$

$$175 \times .80 = 140 \ \text{beats per minute}$$

The training range is 105 to 140 beats a minute.

The chart below will help you to select your target zone. As you can see, maximum heart rate drops with age, so you will need to make adjustments periodically.

Monitoring your pulse takes prior planning, especially if you train on your own—walking briskly, jogging, or riding a stationary bike, for example—and not in a class that includes pulse-taking as part of its program. First, you will need a watch with a second hand; second, you must know in advance what your training range is. After you have been exercising for about five minutes, slow down just enough to focus on the second hand of your watch and take your pulse. Do not stop exercising. Place your fingertips about an inch below your ear at the carotid artery and count the pulse beats for six seconds. (Do not use your thumb; it has a pulse of its own.) Add a zero to the number of beats you counted to get a per-minute rate. If you are over your range, slow your pace; if you are under, increase it; if you are right on, continue exercising for the full 20 to 30 minutes. Eventually, you will feel instinctively what it is like to be within your range and you won't have to bother with this ritual.

If you just can't be inconvenienced with such details, there is another reliable method for determining aerobic status, called the *perceived rate of exertion*. You can easily evaluate your own level of intensity by how heavily you are breathing. If you can't mumble a sound during your workout, chances are you have exceeded the 80-percent range. On the other hand, if you are not panting at all and can recite the Gettysburg Address without missing a beat, accelerate your stride.

There is a wide margin between the low-intensity training rate (60–70 percent) and the high-intensity training rate (70–

Recommended Training Rates

AGE	60%	70%	80%
20	120	140	160
30	114	133	152
40	108	126	144
50	102	119	136
60	96	112	128
70	90	105	120

80 percent), see Figure 6 on page 216. What your rate should be depends on your fitness goals, age, and level of conditioning.

When you exercise within the low-intensity range, your heartbeat is slower and you are not burning as many calories. In some cases this is just the effect you want, because the calories you are burning are from fat only. Fat needs oxygen to burn, and at the lower rate more oxygen is taken in and is available for fat metabolization. As you increase the intensity of the exercise it becomes more difficult to breath deeply, so less oxygen is inhaled. Less fat is burned, and the balance is stored as glycogen; however, you are burning more calories. Each range has its own reward: at low intensity you burn fewer calories but more fat; at high intensity you burn less fat but more calories, which come first from the glycogen supply, then from the muscle.

If you are a beginner, your muscles have probably lost their ability to burn fat, and when you first start out you will be primarily burning sugar.[6] When you go for a walk your muscles will not yet be burning fat, even though you will be breathing heavily for 20 minutes. You may also tire easily and get discouraged when your results are less than you had anticipated. If you are overtired with your workout, cut back and start more slowly. Physical fitness expert Covert Bailey recommends the overweight beginning exerciser not limit her exercising to three times a week. Get out there every day—better yet, two or three times a day—for 10 to 15 minutes, to stimulate your body to initiate the fat-burning process.[7] The untrained body must be constantly introduced to exercise before it starts behaving the way it should. As you become fit, decrease the number of workout days and increase the duration to 20 to 45 minutes.

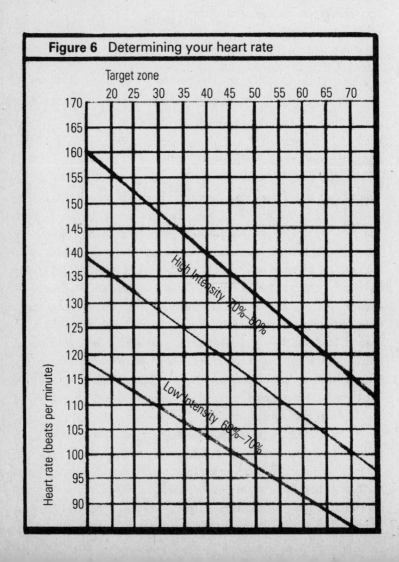

Figure 6 Determining your heart rate

If you have been exercising for a while and you feel your program is no longer working, you may need to give it a boost. Covert Bailey suggests adding intervals of greater intensity throughout your workout so your body can adjust to burning fat at higher levels. By including spurts of intensity in your program your fat-burning potential goes up, and the body learns to be aerobic at levels of exercise that were once anaerobic. (Anaerobic exercise, which means "without oxygen," burns sugar and rapidly leads to exhaustion.) When you are out walking, for example, see if you can work in a few hills, not so difficult that you are gasping for air, but hard enough to make you slightly winded. If you live where there are no hills, you can create the same effect by walking faster for 3 to 5 minutes and then returning to your normal pace.

MUSCLE STRENGTHENING

Adding weight training to an aerobic program offers many benefits to the midlife woman. While strength training doesn't generally reduce body fat, it can help you reverse and rebuild the loss of muscle that comes with natural aging. Several studies suggest that fat mass increases with age while both muscle mass and skeletal mass decline.[8] The reduction in muscle mass eventually leads to the decline in skeletal tissue. Research from the Midlife Center in Gainesville, Florida, found postmenopausal women on hormonal therapy experienced an 8-percent increase in bone mass when they performed muscle-strengthening exercises, while a comparison group of women who took estrogen but didn't exercise neither gained nor lost bone mass.[9] Don't count on hormonal therapy alone to prevent osteoporosis; it is not an alternative to exercise.

Strong, toned muscles protect the joints and help prevent exercise-related injuries. They improve the way your clothes fit and the way you feel about yourself. Women who have not necessarily lost weight but notice definition in their muscles through exercise feel better about themselves.

There are several options for increasing your muscle strength. You can join a club that will introduce you to the proper use of free weights and weight machines like Cybex and Nautilus equipment, or, if you prefer the privacy of your own home, you can purchase your own inexpensive equipment and any number of videos. Some basic exercises are provided in Appendix D. All you need are some 3- to 8-pound dumbbells to build strength in your muscles and bones. Whatever you choose, be sure to get qualified instruction—proper form and technique are essential.

Some women still shy away from weight training and strange-looking machines. Lingering in some women's preconceptions are fears of bulking up or appearing "masculine." Most of us now know that this is a fallacy, because we lack the male hormone, testosterone, that is primarily responsible for male musculature. Using light weights and high repetitions will just firm and strengthen muscles. Using heavier weights and fewer repetitions does build or bulk up more, but not in the same way as it will for a man.

Sometimes, if a woman has a high percentage of body fat (about 28 percent) and starts a muscle-strengthening program before losing some of the fat, she may increase the muscle to a point where the additional muscle along with her body fat makes her look bulky. If you fall in this category, work first on losing some of your weight through reduced fat intake and aerobics, then add a weight-training program.

FLEXIBILITY

The third component of a well-rounded exercise program is flexibility. Muscles and connective tissue lose elasticity with disuse and age. Joints need to move through their full range of motion regularly to maintain flexibility. For many people, one simple form of exercise, stretching, will reduce joint pain and lower-back discomfort, improve posture, and minimize postexercise soreness.

There is a proper way to do everything—even stretching. Stretching should be slow and deliberate to be effective. Rapid or jerky movements are not beneficial and may even be harmful if there is too much tension placed on the muscle being stretched.

It is best to stretch your muscles when they are already warm, so before you start stretching, exercise slowly in the same way you will be using your muscle. For example, warm up for running by jogging slowly; warm up for tennis by swinging your racket. When you warm up, you raise the temperature of your muscles, enabling them to contract more. Stretching before a vigorous workout reduces your chances of being injured, and stretching after a hard workout reduces muscle soreness and enhances muscle relaxation. After exercise your muscles gradually tighten, which reduces flexibility and increases your chances of injury. In summary, before each workout you should warm up and then stretch. After each workout, you should cool down and stretch again.

Stretching, in general, is the best way to increase flexibility and maintain a supple body. An excellent book on the subject is Bob Anderson's *Stretching*. He makes the point that any stretch must be slow and sustained (a minimum of 20 seconds) to be effective.[10] Yoga, too, is excellent for improving flexibility.

THE BOTTOM LINE

Optimal fitness requires more than one kind of exercise. Sheila Cluff from the Oaks at Ojai teaches that there are four major aspects to any fitness workout:

1. A warm-up is very important. You should not shock the body, especially at menopause when it is already coping with many other changes. Move your body gradually from a sedentary mode to an exercise mode. The object is to increase the body temperature, the heart rate, and the muscle demand slowly. Stretching and low-impact exercises, in which the feet stay on the floor, are good warm-up exercises.

2. Next comes the aerobic workout. This doesn't have to be a class; it can be any kind of aerobic activity, but the social support and the music of a class may make it more enjoyable.

3. After the aerobic session, when your muscles are warmed up, work on strengthening all the muscle groups. Don't just concentrate on your "problem" areas; include each and every muscle from your shoulders to your ankles.

4. Cooling down is as essential as warming up. After a hard
    workout, you need to decrease your heart rate and body
    temperature gradually. Stretching will lengthen constricted
    muscles and help the body relieve itself of the toxins and
    lactic acid that have built up. Check your pulse rate again,
    making sure it is back to its normal resting rate.

As you become more physically fit, your resting pulse rate
drops. Most women average around 78 to 84 beats per minute,
while men average 72 to 78. Athletes occasionally drop as low as
35. My resting pulse rate was close to 100 beats per minute before
I started exercising; now it is consistently 55. To get your true
resting pulse rate, take it first thing in the morning before you get
out of bed. Activity, drugs, coffee—almost anything can cause it to
fluctuate. Count the beats for an entire minute; a six-second count
such as you take during aerobics is not sufficient. You can also find
an average resting pulse by taking it several times during the day.
If it stays within a few beats per minute, you are close enough to
have an adequate reading.

As you begin your exercise program, proceed slowly and cautiously. Don't become discouraged; it takes time before results are
noticeable. And don't try to keep up with women who have taken
dance classes since they could walk. Go at your own pace. Excellent guides for beginning aerobic programs are Kenneth Cooper's
The New Aerobics, Covert Bailey's The Fit or Fat Woman, and
Sheila Cluff's Aerobic Body Contouring.

Part Three

NUTRITION FOR LIFE:
A WOMAN'S GUIDE

14

FORMING NEW
EATING HABITS

There is a definite tendency
in our culture towards self-destructive
behavior and living the "good life"
despite dire consequences.
—KENNETH R. PELLETIER, *HOLISTIC MEDICINE*

What we eat and drink every day plays a dynamic role in the way we look, act, and feel. Whether we feel and appear weary or energized, anxious or elated, sickly or fit, is largely determined by our diet. Our future health, how quickly we age, and whether we will succumb to often-fatal degenerative diseases have been proven to be related directly to our dietary lifestyle.

The ancients stressed the importance of good food in health. Some 2,500 years ago, physician-teacher Hippocrates admonished his medical students, "Thy food shall be thy remedy." Today's variation on that axiom is "You are what you eat." Whatever the phrase, the point is that how you feed your body relates directly to your health.

Most of us don't think of nutrition as a separate, complete field of knowledge, but it is. It is a biochemical science based on the incontrovertible laws of nature. When these laws are broken, illness results. A great French physician, Henry Beiler, based his entire practice on the belief that improper foods cause disease and proper foods cure disease. In his famous book *Food Is Your Best*

Medicine, he writes, "Health is not something bestowed on you by beneficent Nature at birth; it is achieved and maintained only by active participation in well-defined rules of healthful living—rules which you may be disregarding every day."[1] Food is not the only factor involved in healthy living, but it is a significant one.

DIET VERSUS DISEASE

It would appear that the American people are not conforming to the rules designed by nature. Despite the abundance of food in the United States, government studies, nutritional surveys, and medical evaluations reveal shocking statistics:

+ Lifestyle (meaning eating and exercise habits) may ultimately account for more than half of all deaths annually in the United States.[2]

+ Current dietary trends may lead to malnutrition through undernourishment.[3]

+ Only 15 percent of women between the ages of 30 and 39 derive less than 30 percent of their calories from fat; only 2 percent get 25 grams of fiber a day.[4]

+ In the US NHANES II data, 41 percent of the population ate no fruit on the survey day; only 25 percent had a fruit or vegetable that contained vitamins A or C.[5]

+ The USDA National Food Consumption Survey showed that only 3 percent of the population eats a "balanced diet." Not a single person of the more than 21,500 surveyed obtained 100 percent of the RDA for all of 10 nutrients listed.[6]

+ Iron deficiency is pervasive in three groups: preschoolers, adolescents, and women over 18.[7]

+ Of women aged 18 to 30 years, 66 percent fail to meet the RDA for calcium; after age 35, the proportion increases to 75 percent.[8]

The good news is that these statistics can be reversed by fairly simple changes in lifestyle. Many of the killer diseases we continually read and hear about (heart disease, arthritis, cancer, and diabetes) have been linked in one way or another to diet and daily habits. Interestingly, these often paralyzing and sometimes fatal conditions have been labeled "diseases of civilization" because of their prominence in rich, industrialized societies that have all the advantages of preserving and processing food.

It is well established that disease related to dietary deficiencies begins far in advance of symptoms. Subtle biochemical changes occur months, even years, before signs wake us up to a potential problem. In the early stages the individual feels nothing out of the ordinary, and medical tests reveal no malfunction. As the disease progresses, there may be generalized symptoms such as fatigue, indigestion, or insomnia. At this point the deficiency may still be difficult to determine, because the clues remain nebulous. Only when serious damage has occurred can a diagnosis be made. Consider the following likely symptoms of nutritional deficiencies. How many sound like menopausal complaints?

Symptoms of Nutritional Deficiencies

✦ low energy

✦ swollen glands

✦ digestive problems

✦ blood disorders

✦ irritability, nervousness

✦ mental problems

✦ insomnia

✦ poor concentration

✦ weight fluctuations

✦ frequent colds and infections

We need to change our frame of reference and concentrate on preventing disease and illness rather than just treating it. For so many life-threatening diseases—osteoporosis, heart disease, and cancer, to name a few—the best and possibly the only real cure is prevention. That voice crying out in the wilderness, out there beyond the "civilized" kingdom of the American Medical Association, is not a quack or an eccentric, but a responsible health professional, the holistic practitioner, saying, "Do something about it *before* it does something to you—before it kills you."

Whether or not you contract a disease depends on more than what you do or do not eat. Your genetic makeup may predispose you to certain illnesses. If your grandmother, mother, sister, or aunt had diabetes, your risk is heightened. Many findings, however, indicate that inherited characteristics exert less influence on our health than the way we live. Not only are there genetic patterns within families, there are also similar dietary habits that may contribute more to the "familial weakness" than genetics. Does your family breakfast on croissants and coffee, lunch on hamburgers, fries, and cola, and dine on steak followed by dessert? You could be in trouble.

Breast cancer, the most common cause of cancer deaths among American women as well as women of other affluent Western countries, is one example of nurture taking precedence over nature. Several studies, including some conducted at the Tufts University School of Medicine and the New England Medical Center in Boston, support the theory that a major determinant for breast cancer in American women appears to be the typical American diet.[9] Studies of disease in cultural populations and other cancer research over the past 20 years seem to confirm that women from Western countries have higher rates of breast cancer than women of most other nations because their diet is low in fiber and high in fat and sugar.

Poor daily habits make you more susceptible to a variety of illnesses. We are all well informed now about the relationships between cigarette smoking and lung cancer, sugar and diabetes, stress and hypertension, cholesterol and heart disease, fiber and digestive disturbances. Whatever we do on a regular basis—whether it is smoking; drinking coffee, cola, or alcohol; eating inordinate amounts of sugar; or working under stress—can promote and provoke very definite and predictable disease states in susceptible individuals.

Diet (and I use the term broadly, to encompass everything that enters the digestive tract, including drinks, drugs, and smoke) may not be the only factor for a healthy body, but it is an extremely vital one. All that you put into your mouth eventually reaches your body's cells, creating the environment in which they grow, replenish, and either thrive or struggle to survive.

WHAT DO HEALTHY PEOPLE EAT?

As part of a search to determine what we should do to become healthy, I have looked into societies and groups of people who have achieved a more optimal state. I found that the most robust people, living the longest number of years, eat foods as varied as the climates from which they come. Laplanders, who live in a bitterly cold climate, eat primarily reindeer meat and suffer none of the degenerative diseases afflicting more prosperous countries. The Polynesians thrive on *poi*, made from the root of the taro plant, raw or cooked fish, and an abundance of fresh tropical plants. The Hunzas of the Himalayas eat mainly whole grains, fresh fruits and vegetables, fresh milk and cheese, and, on occasion, meat, and they are known as the "healthiest people on Earth." In the United States, Mormons show exceedingly low rates of cancer and heart disease. They often grow their own food; eat more cereal, fruit, and vegetables than meat; and refrain from smoking or drinking coffee, tea, or alcohol.

Even though the selections are diverse, there are definite common denominators among the foods eaten by hearty people the world over, and these can help us in determining what we should eat. Weston Price, author of *Nutrition and Physical Degeneration*, found that population groups who live on a natural, unadulterated diet display superb health and freedom from the "diseases of choice" mentioned earlier. When these more "primitive" people adopt modern eating habits, they contract the same degenerative diseases of "civilized" countries within a relatively short period of time (10 years on the average).[10]

The eating habits of healthy peoples, whether they come from the jungles of Africa, the mountains of Tibet, the beaches of the South Pacific, or midtown Manhattan, follow two general rules: Their food is of high nutritional value (what nutritionists call *nutrient dense*), and is unadulterated (not highly processed).

The first component of a nutritious diet is nutrient density. Foods that healthy people consume are loaded with vitamins and minerals in their most natural state. These foods are fresh (locally grown and vine-ripened, and free from pesticides, herbicides, and additives) and raw or lightly cooked. Processed sugars and grains, packaged foods, and commercial additives are generally kept to a minimum.

The bottom line? Eat whole foods (foods that are as near to the way nature created them as possible) and reduce your intake of substitutes that originate in a test tube. This important rule becomes increasingly crucial to our health as we age. With the passing years, cells rebuild more slowly and deteriorate more rapidly. Some nutrients that are not as efficiently absorbed may be required in greater amounts, even though their calories are not. Obviously, we cannot afford to waste our caloric intake on foods that will not feed the body properly.

The foods we consume *most of the time* must be high in nutrient density. We all have favorite recipes, snacks, and celebration delights, and I know you won't deny yourself grandma's famous apple pie forever. As long as these foods are not a daily indulgence, a healthy body will be able to handle them.

For most of us in the United States, our priorities have become reversed over the past 40 years. The balance of what we eat has swung more and more toward nonessential rather than essential foods. It is estimated that up to 80 percent of what the majority of Americans eat has no nutritive value whatsoever. No wonder, then, that the American way of life itself has been called a "high-risk factor" in several diseases. The Senate Select Committee on Nutrition reports that the Standard American Diet (SAD) is high in fat, sugar, and calories, and low in fiber and nutrients. To continue this way of eating when it is *known* to promote high blood pressure, heart disease, digestive disturbances, skin problems, obesity, blood-sugar imbalances, and accelerated aging is indeed

SAD. Several leading nutritionists and the Senate Committee have proposed a more nutritious diet plan (see Figure 7).

If you are at risk for any of the health problems listed above, it is important that you analyze exactly what you are eating. Consider your daily menus: Are the foods you normally eat high in nutrient density? High in fiber? Low in fat? Low in additives (sugar, salt, unnecessary chemicals)? It is also helpful to keep your diet *balanced*, so when you choose your foods, keep the "basic four" nutrition groups in mind (see Figure 8).

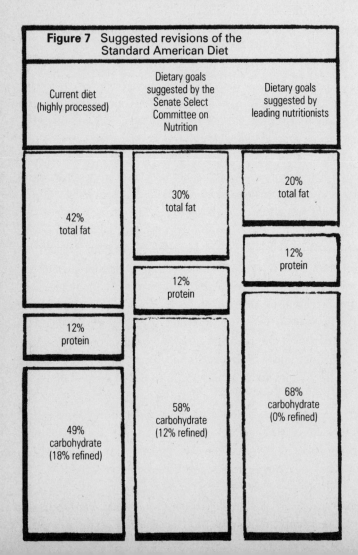

Figure 7 Suggested revisions of the Standard American Diet

Current diet (highly processed)	Dietary goals suggested by the Senate Select Committee on Nutrition	Dietary goals suggested by leading nutritionists
42% total fat	30% total fat	20% total fat
12% protein	12% protein	12% protein
49% carbohydrate (18% refined)	58% carbohydrate (12% refined)	68% carbohydrate (0% refined)

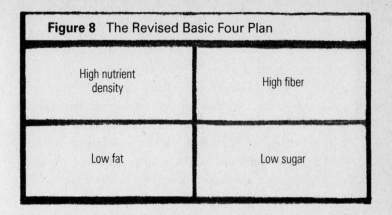

Figure 8 The Revised Basic Four Plan

High nutrient density	High fiber
Low fat	Low sugar

WHEN TO SUPPLEMENT

The question I hear most often when I talk to groups about nutrition is, "Do I need to supplement my diet with additional vitamins and minerals when I normally eat a balanced diet?" My standard answer is, "It depends on your genetic makeup, your diet, your lifestyle, and your individual symptoms." Too often, we lump people into one group, call them average, and proceed to make generalized recommendations on a variety of topics. In the area of health this may not be wise, because we are all different.

If we think in terms of "average" or "normal," we might mistakenly believe that we are receiving adequate nourishment. A better description of the "average" person—if we wish to think of ourselves that way—is found in the authoritative *Heinz Handbook of Nutrition:* "The typical individual is more likely to be one who has average needs with respect to many essential nutrients, but who also exhibits some nutritional requirements for a few essential nutrients which are far from average."

Human beings are not genetically uniform. They vary in body frame, weight, dietary preferences, the amount of exercise they take, their digestion and absorption of nutrients, and how they deal with stress. The nutritional requirements of healthy people can vary from "normal" by a factor of as much as 30; those of sick people may vary by factors as high as 1,000.[11]

This diversity, both biochemical and nutritional, is even greater among women. Consider that some women have no children, some have one child, others have 14. There are women who nurse their babies for several months, women who are on the Pill, women who have had tubal ligations, women who have had partial or radical hysterectomies. Each situation usually requires greater than "average" amounts of specific nutrients. When factors vary so dramatically, it is especially difficult if not impossible to formulate standard or average nutritional requirements.

Many people are born with or develop a need for larger quantities of some nutrients. Andrew Weil, author of *Health and Healing*, explains that our bodies have one or more weak points. Some people are prone to sore throats; others may have sensitive stomachs. Your diet may exacerbate this condition. Nowhere is this clearer than in the case of calcium and its relationship to osteoporosis. Many women inherit a predisposition to osteoporosis; others are at risk because of a lack of calcium in their diet or because of lifestyle habits that prevent calcium absorption. Whatever the case, increased calcium intake can significantly reduce bone loss in the midlife years.

What confuses many people about nutritional recommendations is the fact that there are always stories of individuals who beat the statistics. Why doesn't every smoker get lung cancer when the research so clearly shows a direct correlation between the two? Obviously, some fortunate individuals have strong constitutions, or above-average respiratory systems.

The question you need to ask yourself is not "Am I average?" but "Do I have a weakness?" If so, you should design your diet to compensate for that weakness.

Women tend to be low in iron, calcium, magnesium, zinc, vitamin B-6, and folic acid. Other conditions may indicate greater requirements for certain nutrients. You should consider supplements if you are

+ not eating 2 to 3 fruits and 4 to 5 vegetables a day;

+ drinking excess alcohol, caffeine, or eating sugar;

+ smoking or living with someone who does;

+ on a diet of fewer than 1,000 calories per day;

♦ on a fad diet that restricts a major food group;

♦ pregnant, which usually indicates a need for additional iron and folic acid;

♦ taking medications (diuretics and some hypertensive drugs deplete potassium; cholestyramine causes poor absorption of fat, vitamins A, B-12, and D, and the minerals iron and potassium; mineral oil and other laxatives cause a loss of vitamins A and D and the mineral calcium; and broad-spectrum antibiotics may decrease vitamin K and some of the B-complex vitamins);

♦ diagnosed as having a disease in which diet is a recognized factor: hypertension, heart disease, cancer, kidney disease, ulcers, alcoholism; or

♦ a burn patient, or suffering from a prolonged illness.

If you are a reasonably healthy individual with reasonably healthy parents, a positive outlook on life, and a regular exercise program, and if you maintain your ideal weight, eat a variety of nutrient-rich foods, and avoid excesses of fat, sugar, salt, and alcohol, you probably do not need additional nutrient reserves. On the other hand, if you do have a physiological weakness or a predisposition to a problem, supplements may be a way to fortify your body, improve your vitality, and prolong your life.

15

ACCENTUATE THE POSITIVE

Life is a banquet, but most poor
suckers are starving to death.

— AUNTIE MAME

Nutritionists rarely agree on what constitutes an optimum diet, usually for two reasons: one is that much of nutrition is open to interpretation, and the other, that optimum is different for every individual. Nevertheless, there are certain principles that can be applied when creating an individual program. An optimum diet should allow an individual to develop his or her fullest potential, reach peak mental and physical performance, offer the greatest resistance to infection and disease, and not accelerate the aging process. These goals are widely accepted, so, to start a program, let's fill in the dietary basics that also enjoy general acceptance.

PROTEIN

Eating enough protein is not a problem for most American women, unless they are crash dieting on grapefruit and lettuce leaves. The average protein consumption in the United States substantially exceeds requirements.[1] Believing that a meal must center around meat, many people overdo it. The standard daily requirement of protein is 0.8 grams for every two pounds of your *ideal* body weight. Thus, if you weigh 120 pounds, 48 grams of protein is the amount you need every day to build, repair, and maintain your cells. Women's average intake ranges between 40 and 60 grams per day. The following list translates this into practical measurements.

We all know that protein is basic to life. Next to water, it is the most plentiful substance in the body, constituting 18 to 20 percent of body weight. Protein is the structural material that supports the cells, skin, hair, muscles, internal organs, and blood vessels. It builds cells during times of growth and repairs them in emergencies.

In the United States we have a rather empirical approach to diet. Because we are a

Are You Getting Adequate Protein?

You need: Your body weight in pounds
_____ x 0.4 = _____ grams

FOOD	PROTEIN
beef (8 oz.)	64 g
chicken (8 oz.)	72
fish (8 oz.)	56
tuna (3 oz.)	24
eggs (2)	14
milk (1 cup)	9
cottage cheese (½ cup)	14
cheddar cheese (1 oz.)	7
beans (½ cup)	7
beans with rice (1 cup)	17
vegetarian lasagna (1 cup)	14
rice pudding (1 cup)	17
pasta (1 cup)	5
wheat cereal with milk (1 cup)	28
whole wheat bread (1 slice)	3
cornbread (4" x 3" slice)	4
potato (1, medium)	5

relatively young country with a wide mix of national origins, we do not have a strong "traditional" diet. So we tend to experiment a great deal, trying to sort out the good from the not-so-good. This also means that when something is proven to benefit our health, we have a strong tendency to go overboard. This certainly has happened with protein. For many years, a high-protein diet was the rage. Scores of people suffered dangerous side effects; some even sustained irreversible damage to their organs. Important as protein is to the maintenance of the body, an excess is not beneficial and may even cause serious problems.

For example:

✦ Some meats, especially red meats (beef, pork, lamb) are particularly high in saturated fat. A high-fat diet is known to promote obesity, hypertension, atherosclerosis, and cancer.

✦ Red meats aggravate PMS and menstrual cramps.

✦ Red meats are high in phosphates and acid, which increase the loss of calcium from the bones, creating a greater risk of osteoporosis.

✦ Large amounts of protein put a strain on the kidneys as they form and excrete organic compounds containing nitrogen waste.

✦ Too much protein may deplete vitamins B-6 and B-3, calcium, and magnesium.

✦ Processed and smoked meats such as bacon, ham, salami, and luncheon meats contain nitrates and nitrites, which can lead to the formation of cancer-causing nitrosamines in the body.

Most cuts of meat contain nearly as much fat as protein and possibly even more. A slice of lean ham or a choice grade of slightly marbled sirloin is approximately 25 percent protein and 75 percent fat. Poultry is generally lower in fat and calories, providing, of course, that you remove the skin and don't fry it.

The meat and poultry raised in the United States contain synthetic hormones, antibiotics, pesticide residues, and several other undesirable chemical additives. Fortunately, in some areas of the country poultry products that have been raised untreated are available. Ask about them at your local markets.

Fish is lower in fat than meat and chicken, yet still high in protein. Unless you fry the fish, bread it, or smother it in sauce, the fat content remains low. Of course, it is best to buy fresh fish, but even canned tuna (packed in water), shrimp, and crab are good sources of protein.

Meat, fish, eggs, and all dairy products provide what nutritionists call *complete proteins*. A complete protein contains all eight essential amino acids, or protein building blocks. Protein is also found in varying amounts in vegetables, grains, beans, peas, seeds, and nuts. Because these carbohydrate sources lack or are very low in one or more essential amino acids, they are considered incomplete. Nutritionists used to think that one incomplete protein had to be combined with another incomplete protein at the same meal to get the complete benefit. This theory is no longer accepted since the breakdown fragments of protein, the amino acids, circulate in the body long after a meal is eaten and are easily available for matching.

Though research on proteins and amino acids is fairly recent, cultures all over the world have been combining proteins long before the word was coined. Latin Americans thrive on rice and beans. Corn tortillas and beans are a staple among Mexicans. Traditional dishes in the southeastern United States include corn bread and crowder peas, or red beans and rice. In Chinese cuisine, tofu is added to vegetables and rice. Early vegetarians in the United States have studied the art of food combining to achieve a healthier diet.

Dairy products are not only useful as accompaniments to grains, they are excellent by themselves as a protein source. Milk has been called "the perfect food" because its amino acid balance matches that of meat, fish, and poultry. As with other protein foods, those lowest in fat are preferred: nonfat milk, low-fat cottage cheese, low-fat yogurt, buttermilk, kefir, and cheeses such as mozzarella, bakers' cheese, gammelost, krutt, pot, sapsago, and farmers' cheese. The most popular cheeses—Swiss, cheddar, muenster, longhorn—are highest in fat. Since one ounce of these cheeses contains between 9 and 11 grams of fat, use these sparingly.

Milk is not for everyone, however. Some people are allergic to milk products, and others may lack the enzyme needed to digest the lactose or milk sugar (lactose intolerance). If drinking milk or eating processed cheese causes diarrhea, indigestion, or flatulence, try fermented milk alternatives (yogurt, kefir, buttermilk, or acidophilus milk). If digestive difficulties continue, drop dairy products from your diet. There are enough proteins available from other sources; if you are concerned about your calcium intake, take a supplement.

Seeds and nuts offer another alternative to meat and also double as a good source of fiber. They can be eaten raw and fresh, and can be a convenient snack or combined in a meal for added nutrition, flavor, and texture. Still, power-packed as they are, it is best not to go overboard with these unless you can afford the calories. A half cup of peanuts or walnuts contains 36 grams of fat.

Tofu is close in nutritional quality to meat protein and is an excellent complement to grains. Since tofu is easy to digest and low in saturated fats, cholesterol, and calories, it is recommended for those who cannot eat fat-rich meat and are sensitive to dairy foods.

CARBOHYDRATES

Carbohydrates, supposedly synonymous with weight gain, are shunned by many women. The fact is, once your daily quota of calories has been filled, *any* excess—whether carbohydrates, fats, or proteins—is stored as fat. Thus, all foods are fattening if eaten in excess.

Actually, the body runs on carbohydrates: they are the only true clean-burning fuel in the diet. Both protein and fat release toxic by-products as they are metabolized. Carbohydrates do not; in fact, they temper the toxins. This is why a diet high in protein and fat and low in carbohydrates can overburden the organs and decrease your energy. Athletes and exercise nuts know that carbohydrates are best for fueling the muscles before a workout to protect against muscular fatigue.

Since complex carbohydrates (found in whole grains, beans, rice, fruits, and vegetables) are rich in nutrients, are a great source of fiber, are low in fat, and can double as protein, they can potentially serve our total dietary needs. Vegetarians have long proven that fact. The Senate Select Committee on Nutrition recommends that they constitute the bulk of our diet—60 to 85 percent of our total calories per day.

FIBER

The principal carbohydrates are sugar, starches, and fiber. Sugars and starches basically provide the body with energy, while dietary fiber serves several different functions.

There are several varieties of fiber, and each participates differently in the body. Water-insoluble fiber, found in whole grains and the bran of wheat, rye, corn, and rice, and in some fruits and vegetables, keeps the gastrointestinal system running smoothly. It softens the stool, helps to prevent constipation, and exercises the muscles of the digestive system, keeping the intestines toned and more resistant to diverticulosis.

Soluble fiber is found in high concentration in oat bran, dried peas and beans, barley, and many fruits and vegetables, gums (guar, xanthan, locust bean), mucilages (psyllium), and pectin. A lot of current research proves soluble fiber to be effective in lowering both cholesterol and triglyceride levels in the blood, and in aiding in the regulation of blood-sugar levels.

There is no question that dietary fiber is a major factor in achieving good health. Large-scale research throughout the world suggests that fiber may protect against some forms of cancer, reduce the risk of coronary heart disease, and help control obesity, constipation, diabetes, and a host of other maladies. Fibrous foods also contribute vitamins and minerals to the body. For example, whole-grain flours are rich in B vitamins and protein; fruits give us vitamin C and many minerals; and vegetables are high in vitamin A and minerals.

A quick digression: Let me reemphasize the superior nature of whole grains over processed cereals and breads. In the standard milling process, as much as 60 to 90 percent of vitamin B-6, folic acid, vitamin E, and many other nutrients are lost—as well as the fiber.[2]

Since we generally don't eat enough fruits and vegetables, and since a great deal of the fiber has been processed out of breads and cereals, it is not surprising that fiber intake is abysmally low— less than half of what is considered healthy. Recommended dosage is approximately 30 to 40 grams of fiber per day; most Americans fall below 10 grams per day. Take a quick look at the table on page 238 and see how you score.

You may want to find ways to slowly introduce more fibrous foods into your diet. Adding too many too soon often causes discomfort, so go slowly and work up to at least 30 grams a day.

Suggestions for Increasing the Amount of Fiber in Your Diet

+ Switch to a high-fiber bread, such as sprouted wheat, wheat berry, or 100-percent whole grain.

How Much Fiber Are You Getting?

CEREALS	FIBER
All Bran with extra fiber (1/2 cup)	14.0 g
Wheat Bran (1/2 cup)	12.0
100% Bran (1/2cup)	10.0
Bran Chex (2/3 cup)	6.0
Fruit and Fiber (1/2 cup)	5.0
oatmeal (3/4 cup)	2.1
cornflakes (3/4 cup)	2.1
oat granola (1/3 cup)	1.0
Rice Krispies	0

BREAD	FIBER
pita bread, whole wheat (5" pocket)	4.4 g
100% whole wheat or rye (2 slices)	2.0
bagel (1)	1.4
white bread, French, Italian (1 slice)	0.6
croissant (1)	0

BEANS AND PEAS	FIBER
pinto or kidney beans (3/4 cup, cooked)	14.0 g
black-eyed peas (3/4 cup, cooked)	12.3
garbanzos (3/4 cup, cooked)	7.0
lentils (3/4 cup, cooked)	5.6
split peas (3/4 cup, cooked)	4.0

FRUITS AND VEGETABLES	FIBER
large apple (1)	4.7 g
medium baked potato (1)	4.2
dried apricots (10)	3.6
orange (1)	3.0
cooked corn (1/2 cup)	3.0
peas (1/2 cup)	2.9
carrot (1 raw)	2.3
strawberries (1/2 cup)	2.0
cooked broccoli (1/2 cup)	2.0
medium banana (1)	1.5
peach (1)	1.4
raw spinach (1 cup)	1.4
iceberg lettuce (1 cup)	0.6

+ Have a high-fiber cold cereal for breakfast three to four times a week. Try Bran Flakes, Bran Chex, Raisin Bran, or Cracklin' Oat Bran.

+ Make a high-fiber soup once a week: bean soup, lentil soup, corn chowder, cabbage soup, or vegetable soup with beans.

+ Use beans in your green salads: garbanzo beans, green beans, kidney beans, or peas.

+ Make vegetable dishes that contain beans, such as three-bean salad, succotash, rice with peas, or broccoli with kidney beans.

+ Eat high-fiber vegetables every day, including corn, broccoli, brussels sprouts, spinach, peas, green beans, potatoes.

+ Serve fruit as often as possible, including blueberries, strawberries, pears, raisins, bananas, and apples.

+ Use dark-green salad greens, such as spinach, romaine, and endive, instead of pale iceberg lettuce.

+ Try bean dips served with chili, raw vegetables, or whole-wheat pita bread.

+ Use unprocessed wheat bran and All Bran in regular recipes for pies, cakes, and cookies.

+ Add unprocessed wheat and oat bran to meat loaf, casseroles, and vegetable dishes as an extender, or make crumb toppings for baked fruit desserts.

+ Eat corn, bran, or oat muffins instead of cakes, doughnuts, and cookies.

+ Add raisins to muffins, cereals, rice pudding, and cookies.

+ Use part whole-wheat, soy, or oat flour in your standard recipes.

+ Snack on whole-grain crackers and dried fruits.

+ Use nuts and seeds on salads and in recipes.

FAT

About 40 percent of the calorie intake in the average American diet comes from fats and oils. This is equivalent to about three ounces of fat or three quarters of a stick of butter per person per day. Surprised? Do you trim the fat off your meat, and resist eating bread and butter? Are you convinced someone else—not you—makes up this "average"? The problem is that most of us are unaware of how many fats are camouflaged in our foods. How often do you eat fast foods, TV dinners, deli sandwiches, hot dogs, luncheon meats, peanut butter, bread, crackers, nuts, potato chips, corn chips, avocados, cheese, quiche, salad dressing, pizza, rice pudding, potato salad, paté, pastries, mousse, croissants, dips, doughnuts, ice cream, cheesecake, cream soups, sauces, pie, cookies, and chocolate? These are all high in fat.

A high-fat diet contributes to obesity. Fat has 9 calories per gram compared to 4 calories per gram for both protein and carbohydrates (alcoholic beverages contain 7 calories per gram). A high-fat diet can contribute to the development of high blood pressure, heart disease, diabetes, and breast cancer. Reducing overall fat consumption to 30 percent—or better yet, 20 percent—of your diet should be your long-term goal.

Fats come in many forms, and some are worse for you than others. Two fats in particular, saturated fats and trans fatty acids—earn dishonorable mentions. So, it's best to avoid them. It is also wise to avoid polyunsaturated fats, which are not much better. These fats have been discussed in detail in Chapter 9.

Monounsaturated Fats

These fats are among the few that appear to heal rather than hurt. They include oils like canola, olive, peanut, and sesame, and are your best bet for daily use in salads and cooking. In countries like Greece and Southern Italy, where people take in relatively high amounts of these fats, the rates of heart disease are low.

Essential Fatty Acids

A certain amount of dietary fat is vital to optimum health. Essential fatty acids (EFAs), the fats that we need daily for basic cellular function, are also being recognized for a variety of other therapeutic effects. EFAs have been found to lower cholesterol and blood pressure, to reduce the risk of heart disease and stroke, and, possibly, to be helpful for arthritis and some forms of cancer. They are particularly helpful to midlife women because low levels are partly responsible for drying of the tissues of the body, especially the vagina, skin, and hair.

The essential fatty acids, linoleic acid and linolenic acid, can be found in a variety of sources: raw nuts and seeds, vegetable oils, and fish oils. Getting essential oils through diet is not always easy, since few of us eat large enough amounts of sunflower or pumpkin seeds, or mackerel, salmon, herring, and tuna. Supplementing diet with EFAs is usually indicated for treatment of the conditions mentioned above and may be equally good for preventing problems generally. Recommended sources of EFAs are borage oil, black currant oil, Evening Primrose oil, and flaxseed oil. The last is an excellent source of both EFAs and it can be substituted for other less nutritious oils in salad dressings, mayonnaise, or drizzled on vegetables. To take oils orally as a supplement, 1 to 3 tablespoons daily is adequate. Diabetics should avoid fish oil supplements, but can increase their consumption of fish.

The beneficial effects of EFAs do not mean that you can eat as much of these "healthful" oils as you like. All fats make you fat. Dietary fats are converted more efficiently into body fats than either protein or carbohydrates, and the body expends fewer calories to metabolize them than it does for the other two. If you are concerned about your weight, consume fewer total fats.

Tips for Reducing
Fat Content in Your Diet

+ Cut down on red meats; use them as a side dish rather than as a main course.

+ Buy leaner cuts of red meat, such as round steak, flank steak, and lean ground sirloin.

+ Trim all visible fat from meat before cooking.

+ Replace red meats with turkey and chicken—particularly the white meat.

+ Skin poultry before cooking.

+ Choose fish and seafood more often—especially scrod, flounder, cod, haddock, shrimp, lobster, red snapper, and tuna (packed in water).

+ Bake, broil, or stir-fry rather than deep fry.

+ Experiment with nonmeat dinners once or twice a week.

+ Decrease use of oil and butter in cooking and baking.

+ Minimize cheese, sauces, and dips, and use low-fat substitutes when you can (nonfat milk, low-fat plain yogurt, low-fat cottage cheese).

+ Limit use of seeds, nuts, and avocados.

+ Eliminate processed and packaged foods completely.

+ Watch intake of desserts—especially pies, doughnuts, chocolate, ice cream, and other creamy, gooey concoctions. (Try substituting nonfat desserts instead.)

WATER

Water is an often overlooked ingredient in the good health and energy equation. Next to oxygen it is the most important nutrient we can give our bodies. A healthy adult can survive for weeks without food, but only days without water. A loss of even 10 percent of total body fluid is serious.

Water is essential to all living organisms. It is the major constituent of body fluid, making up about half of the body weight in an average adult female and about 60 percent in the adult male. This percentage varies inversely with the fat content of the body: when less fat is present, water is a greater percentage of the body weight.

Water is absolutely essential to blood building and internal cleansing, to the proper functioning of the kidneys and sweat glands, and the entire digestive process. It facilitates the transportation of nutrients and hormones to the cells and flushes toxic wastes from the body. People who drink a lot of water seldom have elimination problems.

In addition to transporting molecules of oxygen and hydrogen to the cells, water is also, in itself, a source of minerals that are particularly important to the blood, bones, and heart. Several studies in both the United States and the United Kingdom have found that rates of death from heart disease are generally lower in regions where people drink mineralized "hard" water. Soft water may be great for laundry, but its lack of calcium and magnesium in addition to its high sodium content make it a poor choice for drinking.

Many people mistakenly feel they are consuming their quota of liquid because they continually drink coffee, tea, soft drinks, and diet drinks. Even though these beverages are water based, the pure water has been corrupted with syrup, caffeine, and chemical additives. Instead of hydrating the system, these draw the water out; instead of cleansing, they pollute and burden the dried-out organs; instead of quenching, they cause thirst.

As we age, we naturally lose about 10 to 15 percent of our body fluid. If we compound this loss by continually dehydrating our bodies with coffee, sugar, and alcohol, we are likely to wrinkle and age prematurely. For moist mucous membranes on the inside and plump-looking, wrinkle-free skin on the outside, we must drink a lot of fresh water.

Certain foods contain a great deal of water and are refreshing, cleansing, and energizing. More than 90 percent of juicy fruits and vegetables such as tomatoes, lettuce, cauliflower, eggplant, watermelon, and strawberries are water. Whole milk is 87 percent water; avocados, bananas, and sweet potatoes contain 75 percent water; and, strangely enough, many kinds of low-fat fish are a fair source of water.

However, we cannot depend on foods to fill our need for fluid. Persons of average build should drink six to eight 8-ounce glasses of pure spring or bottled water each day—more if it is hot, if they are exercising, if they are having hot flushes, and (believe it or not) if they are bloated or retaining water.

The foods we eat and the fluids we drink all work together in creating good health. High-quality proteins and fibrous carbohydrates low in saturated fat provide the raw materials necessary for a healthy body.

16

Eliminate the Negative

Every day you do one of two things:
build health or produce disease in yourself.
—ADELLE DAVIS

NONFOOD ADDITIVES

To choose healthful foods, look for those that are as close to their original, whole state as possible. This means avoiding foods whose natural integrity has been violated. Foods created in a laboratory cannot match the nutritional quality of a natural product. Even if they have been carefully designed to incorporate several vitamins and minerals, they do not contain the mysterious micronutrients—enzymes and trace minerals—that have yet to be discovered and duplicated. For these elusive elements, we need "real" food. This is why most nutritionists prefer foods to pills as the source of nutrients.

Almost all reports and research indicate that the health and longevity of a population are related to the naturalness and wholesomeness of the foods they eat. In cultures where the diet consists totally of fresh, whole, unprocessed, and unrefined foods, people (if they get enough to eat) enjoy good health, long life, and a relative absence of disease. Once their diet changes to include denatured, refined, human-made foods, disease creeps in and people lose their mysterious secret of life and good health.

Virtually all supermarket food today contains chemicals that were added either in the growing stage or during processing. Long before most foods reach manufacturers, they are treated with fertil-

izers, herbicides, and pesticides; injected with hormones, tranquilizers, and antibiotics; or exposed to the chemical wastes of industrial
society. In a survey released in April 1994, the USDA found residues of 49 different chemicals in 61.2 percent of the apples, bananas, carrots, celery, grapes, grapefruit, oranges, peaches, lettuce,
and potatoes. Of these, about 1 percent had residues above the
legal limits set by the Environmental Protection Agency.[1] Apples
had the highest pesticide findings, with 88.5 percent of those sampled containing at least one residue.

As a food is prepared and packaged it may be treated with a
number of additional chemicals, some of which may be harmful.
For example, a group of acknowledged carcinogens—sodium nitrate and sodium nitrite—are routinely used to preserve luncheon
meats, hot dogs, smoked fish, bacon, and ham. There is no question that these additives produce a cancer-causing substance, yet
they continue to be used—supposedly in quantities small enough
to be harmless.

To list all the pollutants and poisons found in processed foods
would take a book in itself. There are literally thousands, disguised
as stabilizers, imitation flavors, thickeners, softeners, emulsifiers,
sweeteners, bleaches, enhancers, conditioners, ripeners, waxes,
acidifiers—and the list goes on. Yet many research studies show
that when taken together, interacting, they may not be harmless at
all, and that we—or the manufacturers—may be playing Russian
roulette with our lives and health. It may shock you to know that
each of us supposedly consumes about 5 pounds of these additives
per year. The long-term effects of many of them are still unknown,
as are the cumulative consequences of a lifetime of ingesting these
substances.

The food industry determined long ago that these substances
are necessary to maintain shelf life, to preserve the appearance, or
to enhance the appeal of a product. There is little chance it will
stop using them in the interest of better nutrition. Large-scale
production has always been motivated more by profits than health.
As consumers we have two choices: we can vow never to eat a
food that has been "adulterated" (eliminating just about everything
at the grocery store), or we can be prudent in our selection of
products, taking the time to read and compare labels. In time, if

enough consumers select foods with fewer additives, the food industry will respond and start reducing, perhaps even eliminating,
the additives. One more safeguard is to eat a variety of foods,
reducing the risk of getting too much of a particular additive.

If it is available, look for produce that is organically cultivated, food that is grown without the aid of pesticides and herbicides. Sixteen states have adopted laws governing organic food and
farming practices: California, Colorado, Iowa, Maine, Massachusetts,
Minnesota, Montana, Nevada, New Hampshire, North Dakota,
Ohio, South Dakota, Texas, Vermont, Washington, and Wisconsin.
These laws ensure that no harmful pesticides or herbicides are used
on the soil or on the produce. Organic fruits and vegetables are
widely available in specialty markets, health food stores, and local
farmers' markets, and are slowly infiltrating major market chains. If
everyone would start asking their local grocery store manager
about incorporating more organically grown foods in the inventory,
we would have a greater selection and, hopefully, prices would
come down. If you have no choice in the matter and are forced to
purchase conventionally grown produce, wash it well in a mild
additive-free soap, or peel off the skin and remove the outer layers.

SUGAR

Two food additives deserve special mention because they are so
terribly overused in the western diet. Since both sugar and salt are
relatively inexpensive, they are used extensively to preserve, flavor,
and extend the shelf life of many products. If you think your diet
is relatively low in sugar, go into your pantry and read the labels.
Sugar, disguised in its many different forms as dextrose, sucrose,
fructose, maltose, corn syrup, beet sugar, honey, and molasses, probably appears on all your product labels: canned fruits and vegetables,
yogurt, salad dressing, pickles, catsup, antacids, and cough medicine.
Many items contain more than one form of sugar, so be assured
you are getting better than your fair share. Believe it or not, most
Americans individually consume 140 pounds of sugar per year.

As we approach menopause, we require fewer calories but the
same amount of nutrients. We need to minimize foods that not
only lack nutritive value but also destroy the nutrients we have

consumed. Sugar is at the top of the list. How bad is it? So bad that not even a lowly microbe can survive in it.

As sugar is metabolized, it drains the body of many vitamins. Unlike natural carbohydrates—such as apples, oranges, and whole grains—refined white sugar enters the body unaccompanied by the team of nutrients needed to facilitate its digestion and assimilation. These nutrients are leached out of the body's resources. Over time, this creates multiple deficiencies, especially within the B-complex family. As a result, most women with a sweet tooth are deficient in B vitamins. Initial signs of such deficiency are relatively minor: fatigue, water retention, anxiety, irritability, and depression. Long-term deficiencies, however, may have serious consequences. Studies at McGill Medical School have determined that there is a direct correlation between B-vitamin deficiency and estrogen-based cancers.[2] In the absence of adequate B vitamins, estrogen builds up and is subsequently stored in the estrogen receptors of the breast and uterus. A vicious cycle results: as the production of estrogen increases, the deficiency becomes more pronounced; the greater the deficiency, the more estrogen is secreted.

Sugar significantly alters the levels of several hormones as they attempt to maintain a chemical balance within the body. The pancreas, liver, and adrenal glands are all overstimulated by fluctuation in blood-sugar levels. While our bodies can handle blood-sugar highs and lows in our youthful years, the day of reckoning comes when our systems loses their resilience.

For menopausal women, symptoms of this change may be related to the inability of the worn-out adrenal glands to take over estrogen production as the ovaries decline. When the glands are strong and healthy, they are much more capable of secreting the amounts of estrogen needed to prevent dramatic hormonal fluctuations, which are related to menopausal symptoms.

Probably the most critical problem women face, both before and during menopause, is getting and absorbing enough calcium to prevent osteoporosis. Sweet eaters beware! Sugar inhibits calcium absorption. To guard against the most devastating of all menopausal problems—brittle bones—watch your sugar *now*.

A sweet tooth, like any bad habit or addiction, can be brought under control if one is truly motivated. For some women, conscious awareness is enough to make the change. Women who have become physically addicted to sugar may actually experience withdrawal symptoms when it is eliminated. Approach the change with care, planning, self-love, and patience. Retraining your taste buds will take time and effort. Don't try to reverse 30 years of indiscriminate eating in two days, or two weeks.

Everyone asks for advice on how to handle sugar cravings. I recommend that you concentrate on the specific micronutrients affected by eating sugar: the B vitamins, magnesium, chromium, zinc, and manganese. Foods rich in these substances include certain fruits and vegetables, whole grains, and wheat germ. But don't wait until you have given in to the desire for a double hot-fudge sundae to start suddenly eating greens. Prepare your body in advance by keeping it well nourished and well supplied.

Artificial sweeteners are not the best alternative to sugar, although they may be temporarily useful. Saccharine, cyclamates, and aspartame have all been linked to cancer and have various side effects. To replace one potential enemy with another is hardly satisfactory. What we ultimately must do is to retrain the expectation of our taste buds for sweetness.

You are probably wondering about the value of raw sugar, molasses, carob, and honey—the so-called natural sugars. Bad news: all forms of sugar, in the amounts we normally eat them, deplete the nutrient supply and cause a sudden elevation in the blood sugar. Unlike table sugar or sucrose, however, these more respected natural sweeteners do have some nutritional value: carob is rich in B vitamins and minerals; honey contains small amounts of trace minerals and traces of the vitamins B, C, D, and E; molasses is high in iron, calcium, copper, magnesium, phosphorus, and vitamins B and E. If you must use a sweetener for baking or on your cereals, the natural ones are slightly better. Just use them sparingly.

Why Women Must Control Their Cravings for Sweets

+ Sugars are nonnutritive.

+ They deplete vitamin and mineral stores, especially vitamins B and C and the minerals magnesium and chromium.

+ They create hormone fluctuations and imbalances, aggravating menstrual problems.

+ They cause extremes in blood-sugar levels.

+ They create severe stress in the endocrine glands (adrenals, pancreas).

+ They trigger hot flashes.

+ They inhibit calcium absorption, and thus can contribute to osteoporosis.

+ They are addictive.

+ They have been linked to obesity, digestive disturbances, tooth decay, diabetes, increased blood cholesterol and triglyceride levels, and urinary tract infections.

SALT

Table salt, or sodium chloride, has been used for a long time to preserve food. Unlike simple sugar, however, sodium is an essential nutrient. It is required for the maintenance of blood volume, the regulation of fluid balance, the transport of molecules across cell walls, and the transmission of impulses along nerve fibers.

Recent government studies indicate, however, that most Americans consume far more table salt than they need. Even when no salt is added during cooking or at the table, the sodium quickly adds up. We take in daily, on the average, between 6 and 20 grams of sodium chloride; we need no more than 1 to 3 grams per day. This is no more than is found in the foods we normally eat.

Eating too much salt can raise the blood pressure and increase the risk of heart and kidney disease. Salt stimulates water retention, which is uncomfortable, adds unwanted pounds to the body, and prevents the loss of fat. In the menopausal woman, salt may trigger annoying hot flashes and promote loss of calcium from the bones. The exact amount of calcium loss and bone breakdown caused by high salt intake is not known, but any loss is significant for high-risk women in their middle years.

Sodium can also aggravate premenstrual syndrome. Niels Lauersen writes that eliminating salt from their diet alone has helped many PMS sufferers reduce their bloatedness, premenstrual irritability, and headaches.[3] He indicates that it is especially important for women with PMS to reduce their salt intake during the two weeks preceding their periods, when PMS symptoms can be the worst.

To reduce salt in your diet, start with the obvious offenders: chips, crackers, ham, bacon, other smoked or cured meats, processed cheese, and table salt. Then look for the hidden salt in processed foods. In checking labels, look for anything with the word *sodium* in it, such as monosodium glutamate and sodium nitrate, and watch for the abbreviated chemical symbol for sodium, *Na*.

Sodium Content of Common Foods

eggs (2, medium)	108 mg
ground beef (¼ lb.)	76
hamburger (1 commercial)	950
hot dog	627
haddock (4 oz.)	201
whole-wheat bread (1 slice)	148
corn flakes (½ cup)	126
waffle	356
chocolate cake (1 piece)	233
fresh peas (½ cup)	2
canned peas (½ cup)	200
potato (1 medium)	6
hash brown potatoes (½ cup)	223
milk (1 cup)	128
low-fat cottage cheese (1 cup)	918
cheddar cheese (1 oz.)	176
roquefort cheese (1 oz.)	513
dill pickle	928
commercial salad dressing (1 Tbsp.)	219
canned minestrone soup (1 cup)	2,033

Commonly available salt substitutes contain potassium in place of all or part of the sodium. People under medical supervision, particularly for kidney problems, should check with their physicians before using salt substitutes. Alternatives that contain mixtures of spices and herbs, such as Veg-It, may be better choices. You can also substitute mixed herbs, fresh spices, garlic, lemon juice, and unsalted salad dressing. Be creative, find new tastes you like, and experiment with them. Once you do, you will find it difficult to eat something that is highly salted. Many good books have also been written with excellent recipes for a low-salt diet. My favorite is *The American Heart Association Cookbook*.

You should also be cautious of what you drink. Soft water, carbonated soda, and some bottled waters contain sodium. Ordinary club soda has 241 mg; Perrier water, 14 mg; and Poland Spring water, 4 mg. This may be more important if you are prone to PMS, water retention, or high blood pressure.

CAFFEINE

Coffee is the most widely used stimulant in the United States. Hidden behind the friendly color and delicious aroma of brewing coffee is the stimulant drug, caffeine. This white crystalline alkaloid produces strong physiological effects, some of which we know and desire, and others about which we are uninformed. Caffeine stimulates the central nervous system, warding off fatigue and temporarily giving us the feeling of mental alertness. In some individuals it may create a general sense of well-being, improve reaction time, enhance accuracy, and even enhance endurance. But that is only half the story.

When caffeine is taken in excess—and that limit is a function of individual tolerance—the entire central nervous system is overstimulated. Nervous reactions that result may include shakiness, heart palpitations, chronic anxiety, and dizziness. Menopausal women report that caffeine often triggers hot flashes, sweating, and insomnia.

Caffeine promotes the release of insulin from the pancreas and of adrenalin from the adrenal cortex, raising the blood-sugar level initially to an unnatural high, which soon drops to an unhealthy low. Contrary to the hopes and dreams of dieters, the insulin response initiated by the stimulant winds up increasing the appetite, enhancing the craving for sweets and encouraging the storage of fat.

An effective diuretic, coffee forces the excretion of more than normal amounts of water, vitamins, and minerals. The water-soluble vitamins B and C are particularly susceptible to forced water loss. Calcium can also be lost by drinking too much coffee.

Caffeine has been implicated in the development of fibrocystic breast disease. Eliminating caffeine completely has been shown to reduce both the size and painfulness of the cysts in two to six months.[4] As both a coffee lover and a woman with fibrocystic breast pain, I can confirm the results of this research. Only one small latte will give me pains within the hour, and forget espresso.

Caffeine affects the gastrointestinal, cardiovascular, and circulatory systems as well. Shortly after you drink a cappuccino, your stomach temperature rises, your hydrochloric acid output increases, your heart beats faster, and the blood vessels constrict (narrow) around the brain, yet dilate (widen) around your heart. Your metabolic rate increases, the uric acid in your blood increases, the blood flow to your extremities is reduced, and your eyeball pressure is raised. Anyone suffering from glaucoma should be warned against drinking coffee.

Determining Caffeine Levels

SOURCE	MILLIGRAMS
coffee (1 cup)	
drip	110–150
percolated	64–124
instant	40–108
tea (1 cup)	
black, brewed 5 min.	20–50
black, brewed 1 min.	9–33
instant	12–28
iced	22–36
soft drinks (12 oz)	
Coke	46
Pepsi	41
Tab	46
Mountain Dew	54
Diet Coke	46
chocolate	
milk chocolate (1 oz.)	20–35
hot chocolate (1 cup)	5–10
medications	
Excedrin	65
(Excedrin P.M. has no caffeine)	
Anacin	32
Midol	32
Cope	32
Dexatrim	200
No Doz	100
Darvon	32
Vivarin	100
aspirin	0

The effects of caffeine are systemwide, touching every organ, tissue, and cell in the body. Caffeine has also been linked to the incidence of several cancers; however, more studies are needed to confirm these reports.

A "moderate" dose of caffeine is 2 mg per pound of body weight; thus, if you weigh 130 pounds, it is considered "safe" for you to take in 260 mg of caffeine per day. This isn't very much when you consider that a single cup of coffee contains between 100 and 150 mg of caffeine. Remember, too, that coffee is not the only common source of caffeine, which is a major ingredient in many over-the-counter diet pills and in prescription drugs for pain, menstrual cramps, allergies, and headaches. Use the following list to determine how much caffeine you may be taking into your body.

Changing any lifelong pattern can be stressful. Most experts suggest a gradual process for weaning yourself off coffee, rather than stopping cold turkey. Because caffeine is a drug, when you stop abruptly you may experience withdrawal symptoms: headaches, drowsiness, nausea, nervousness, depression, indigestion, edema, constipation, cramps, and, strangely, even a runny nose. Give yourself time to make this transition. Taper off by eliminating a few cups a day if you are a heavy coffee drinker. Substitute with decaffeinated coffee some of the time, or try tea or, better yet, herb tea, Postum, juice, mineral water, or plain water with a twist of lemon. Once you have kicked the coffee habit, you will have more natural energy than you did after your four-cup fix.

ALCOHOL

Alcohol provides little or no nutrition, depletes vital nutrients, and places a heavy burden on the hormonal system, the digestive system, and the kidneys. Taken to extremes, alcohol consumption actively damages organs such as the pancreas and the liver, and can disrupt the entire nervous system permanently. It increases the risk of diabetes, heart disease, and cancer; and its addictive qualities are, for some people, a nightmare.

Certain women are hypersensitive to alcohol. PMS sufferers have a lowered alcohol tolerance during the days preceding their periods. Even one glass of wine may be enough to cause intoxication.

The potential long-term effects of alcohol consumption are even more frightening. One British study indicates that women who drink regularly have a 1.5 to 2 times higher rate of breast cancer than those who never drink.[5] Women who both smoke and drink are at even greater risk, suggesting that there may be multiple adverse factor in effect when both habits are involved.

One explanation for why alcohol may increase the risk of breast cancer is proposed by nutritional biochemist Jeffrey Bland. He believes that it is related to the adverse effect alcohol has on the liver. One function of the liver is to break down estrogen so that it can be excreted safely from the body. "The inability to properly metabolize estrogen can lead to the buildup of certain estrogenic substances within the body that can overly stimulate receptors in the breast, ovary, or uterine wall and initiate a cancer process."[6] As was noted previously, B vitamin deficiencies can also cause estrogen oversecretion, and alcohol depletes B vitamins.

Over half of the problems associated with excessive long-term alcohol consumption stem from the malnutrition that results from continual use. Alcohol, a derivative of sugar, is metabolized in the body in a similar way. It requires substantial nutrients from other sources or from the body's reserves before it can be metabolized, or converted into energy. Thus, it creates deficiencies of the B vitamins, vitamin C, calcium, magnesium, potassium, and zinc.

Any woman at risk for osteoporosis should carefully monitor her alcohol intake. Alcohol impairs calcium absorption and may affect the ability of the liver to activate vitamin D. It is not known how much alcohol it takes to effect significant bone loss; what has been established, though, is the fact that alcoholics are at much greater risk for developing osteoporosis.

Alcohol has also been reported to aggravate the common menopausal symptoms of hot flashes, insomnia, and depression. Since it is high in calories, it easily adds unwanted pounds around the midsection. And as a dehydrant, alcohol, in excess, can result in premature wrinkling and loss of skin tone.

Individuals who eat healthy diets and are in good physical condition can take the occasional drink without serious detrimental effects; it may even have some health benefits. Alcohol in moderation is a social lubricant. It can relieve tension, stimulate the appetite (aperitif), and aid digestion (digestif). As I have said, it is not what you eat or drink *occasionally* that will harm you; it's what you put into your body on a regular basis.

Recent reports have indicated that one or two ounces of alcohol a day may slightly decrease the risk of heart disease by increasing high-density lipoproteins—the fraction of cholesterol that seems to protect against atherosclerosis. I do not advocate drinking alcohol in order to raise your HDLs, however; exercise is every bit as effective and has no side effects.

To a large degree, alcohol tolerance is an individual—or family—matter. If you are hypoglycemic; have a history of breast cancer in your family; are prone to osteoporosis; suffer from hot flashes, depression, insomnia, or PMS; or have a problem with moderate drinking; you probably need to refrain from alcohol completely.

CIGARETTES

Smoking is the largest single cause of premature death and ill health for women and men in America. A woman who smokes runs twice the risk of dying from stroke, and 8 to 12 times the risk of dying from lung cancer. Because women are now smoking as much as men, they have caught up with men in incidence of lung cancer, and it is now the number one cancer killer of women, exceeding even breast cancer.

The risks of smoking increase with age and the number of years one has been smoking. They include osteoporosis, glaucoma, cardiovascular disease, and several kinds of cancer. There is an increased risk of heart disease among women who both take oral contraceptives and smoke, and an increased risk of cancer of the mouth, pharynx, larynx, and esophagus among people who both smoke and drink.

A wonderful book that addresses the reasons women smoke and the unique difficulties—physiologically and psychologically—they have quitting is *How Women Can Finally Stop Smoking,* by Dr. Robert Klesges and Margaret DeBon.

17

Putting Your Diet into Action

Knowing is not enough; we must
apply. Willing is not enough;
we must do.

—GOETHE

What we eat and how we live in our younger years directly determines the quality of our future health. For this reason, we need to analyze our eating habits and see if we are adequately prepared.

As we get older, it becomes increasingly important to monitor the quality of food we eat. Physical problems increase because the body cannot produce hormones, enzymes, and antibodies at the same rate and in the same amounts as before. Nutrients are absorbed and used less efficiently. To maintain health, we must provide the body with a steady supply of high-grade nutrients, and avoid foods and substances that strain the system.

For some this may mean embarking on a major program to take charge of their health. The first steps are determining where you are and what you want to accomplish. Awareness of the need to change always precedes action, and you should take some time now to understand your individualized needs. Before you make any specific dietary alterations, or go out and spend a fortune on supplements, first analyze your eating habits, your lifestyle, and your present symptoms.

CHARTING FOR HEALTH

Prior to taking action, check any and every unusual symptom with your family doctor. Even something as seemingly innocuous as fatigue could indicate a serious problem. When you have a clean bill of health, then proceed.

Any new program must begin with the basics, and that is precisely where we will start, with the most basic substance our body needs: good, wholesome, nutritious food. The first step is to review everything that enters your mouth. The most effective way to do this is by charting—writing down every day, for several weeks, exactly what you eat and drink.

You could use a very large calendar, such as a desk calendar, or buy some poster paper and make your own chart. This will also reinforce your serious intent to change your habits. Now, write down your eating patterns for three weeks. Why so long? For several reasons: It is important to record and review different eating situations, such as weekend parties, family get-togethers, lunches out, office meals, and days alone. It is especially important to analyze the week before, during, and after your menstrual period.

The same kind of dieting chart illustrated in Chapter 1 and used in gaining control of your weight is excellent for helping you gain control of your nutrition. Make three columns: a narrow one for the times of day you eat or snack, a wider one for the food, and another narrow one for recurring feelings or symptoms. Be specific when you fill it in—for example, write down the *kind* of cereal (oatmeal, cornflakes, or bran flakes), the *kind* of bread (white, rye, whole-grain wheat), *how* the food was prepared (fried, broiled, steamed, raw), and how *much* you ate. Don't forget condiments: catsup, mustard, mayonnaise, pickles, and so on. In the symptom column, record how you feel; you can use your own system of abbreviations or symbols. Fill in this column as and when your symptoms occur—midmorning, after lunch, and so on.

After a very interesting—and revealing—three weeks, you will be ready for the dietary and lifestyle test below. It might be easier if you go through your chart and circle specific areas with different colored pens (e.g., sugar foods with red, fatty foods with green, and processed foods with blue). After three weeks have gone by, you will definitely be in touch with your eating habits. Not only will you know the types of foods you eat regularly, but you will also see how often you eat (or don't eat) and how frequently you experience recurring symptoms.

As a cross-check or a quick self-test, you can get a general idea of your dietary habits right now. In the questionnaire below put a check next to each item for which your answer is yes.

Dietary and Lifestyle Analysis

1. Do you frequently (more than 4 times a week) eat
    __ fast foods
    __ canned fruits, vegetables, and soups
    __ fried, breaded, or deep-fried meats or vegetables
    __ desserts, doughnuts, cupcakes, cookies, pie, ice cream
    __ packaged or frozen foods, instant products
    __ white bread, white rice
    __ hot dogs, bacon, luncheon meats
    __ chips and crackers
    __ condiments (catsup, mustard, syrups, jam, mayonnaise)
    __ candy

2. Do you frequently drink
    __ coffee, more than 2 cups a day
    __ soft drinks, diet drinks, tea, decaffeinated coffee
    __ alcohol, more than 5 times a week

3. Do you often skip one or more meals?

4. Are you on a diet of fewer than 1,000 calories per day?

5. Do you smoke?

6. Do you take medication?

7. Are you continually under stress?

8. Are you inactive, having no regular exercise program?

9. Do you have several annoying symptoms (gas, fatigue, headaches, hemorrhoids, insomnia)?

If you checked fewer than five items, your diet is probably healthful. If you checked close to half, you need to make some adjustments in your diet or life-style. If you checked most of the items, you should get a physical and reevaluate your lifestyle. You definitely need both a drastic change of diet and nutritional reinforcement.

ARE YOU DEPRIVING YOUR BODY OF NUTRIENTS?

Your next step is to determine whether or not your daily habits are diminishing your vitamin and mineral supply. Many people do not realize the serious consequences environmental forces, drugs, and their own daily habits can have in terms of nutritional deficiencies. Some factors, such as the air we breathe, are unavoidable; some, such as medications and stress, can be controlled somewhat; and many, such as sugar, salt, and fat consumption, are completely within our power to change. The ideal is to avoid as many of these poor habits as possible. If you are not ready to give up your favorite vice, the least you can do is fortify the body so your overall health will not be compromised.

How many of these items are a part of your life? Circle them. What nutrients might you be compromising? Do they appear more than once? Twice? Refer to your daily chart. Are you eating foods that supply these nutrients? For example, if you smoke, eat a lot of cooked and frozen foods, lunch meats, and bacon (high in nitrates), and take medications like aspirin or Indocin, you may require additional vitamin C. Keeping this in mind, check your chart again. How many foods do you eat that are high in vitamin C? If you are not eating fresh fruits and vegetables every day, you need to consider adding them to your diet or taking vitamin C supplements.

Once you have analyzed your dietary habits, you are ready to make some changes. Whatever you do, don't try to tackle all your problems in the first week. You will just give up in frustration. Choose one area that you want to work on; when you feel that is under control, go for another.

You may not feel immediate improvement, but after a few months you should notice subtle changes: an increase in energy, less stomach distress, a clearer mind, more radiant skin and hair, stronger nails, easier and shorter menstrual periods, a sense of well-being, and a feeling of calmly energetic good health. I have experienced it, and I have seen it happen to many others. A healthier diet and lifestyle will reward you in ways you cannot imagine.

READING YOUR BODY

Don't trash your new chart yet, even if you feel you know all about your eating patterns. There is a third column, remember? Symptoms. What are yours? Do you have a lot of those "normal" complaints? Are you run down? Do you have the Monday morning droops? The afternoon slump? The blahs? Are you tired? Listless? Have "female problems"? Cramps? The premenstrual crazies? Read on.

Many people suffer from marginal nutrient deficiencies. They are not what you would call sick—that is, they don't have anything with a Latin-sounding name. A marginal deficiency is "a condition of gradual vitamin or mineral depletion in which there is evi-

Vitamin and Mineral Depleters

DEPLETER	NUTRIENT DEPLETED
caffeine	B-complex, especially thiamine (B-1); inositol, potassium, zinc
alcohol	B-complex, C, A, magnesium, zinc
sugar	B-complex, chromium, zinc, manganese
high-fat/protein diet	calcium
refining process	B-complex, many minerals
crash dieting	A, B-complex, C, D, E, calcium, zinc, potassium
chlorinated water	E
inorganic iron	E
cigarettes	A, C, E, calcium, selenium
pollution	A, C, E, selenium
stress	B-complex, C, zinc, all nutrients
infection	A, B-complex, C, E, zinc
cooking	A, B-complex, C
freezing	C, E
nitrites	A, C, E
ERT	E, zinc, magnesium
aspirin	C, folic acid, pyridoxine (B-6)
antibiotics	B-complex, C, K, potassium
antacids	thiamine (B-1), phosphorus
antihistamines	C
barbiturates	A, C, D, folic acid
cortisone	A, pyridoxine (B-6), C, D, zinc, potassium
Indocin	thiamine (B-1), C
laxatives/ diuretics	A, D, E, K, potassium

dence of lack of personal well-being associated with impaired physiological function."[1] Roughly translated, that means: you can feel that something is out of sync, but tests don't reveal any major functional problem.

The body operates on a fresh and continuing supply of nutrients. When these are missing for an extended period of time, functions deteriorate, setting off a series of reactions that begin subtly at the cellular level and gradually move up to the tissue and organ level. Initially, the body compensates for deficiencies by using stored nutrients. Some nutrients, however, cannot be stored for more than one day, and, in time, the stores of others get seriously low. Examples of these are the B vitamins and vitamin C.

Myron Brin, Ph.D., a nutrition researcher at Hoffman–La Roche (a pharmaceutical firm) and one of the pioneers in this area, has identified consecutive phases of marginal deficiencies in the body. In the preliminary stage, nutrients stored in the body's tissues are gradually depleted, because of low intake, poor absorption, or abnormal metabolism. At this point there are no symptoms or detectable physical signs. As deficiencies progress to the biochemical stage (the stage at which changes can be detected through chemical tests), tissue stores are depleted. There are still no obvious clues, but silent destruction is occurring beneath the surface of the skin. Even though nothing can be detected on the outside, the tissue damage can have a significant effect on functions such as the body's ability to handle drugs, alcohol, or exposure to environmental chemicals, and its immunity to disease.[2]

Clues start appearing only in the final stage, where they show up as behavioral and psychological manifestations. Nonspecific symptoms such as loss of appetite, depression, anxiety, or insomnia may be among the first signals that you are undernourished. If you notice yourself writing these symptoms in several entries on your daily chart, consider it a warning of marginal nutrient deficiencies.

In the final stages definite clinical signs appear and, if left untreated, eventually result in disease. Of course this is what we want to avoid and, to a certain degree, can, by heeding our bodies' subtle, nonspecific signals before they reach a critical point.

Most bodily reactions involve several biochemical pathways or steps. Several nutrients, enzymes, and hormones may be required for one particular organ system to function. A shortage of just one vitamin can result in a collection of different symptoms involving the skin, hair, eyes, mouth, or teeth, or the digestive, muscular, nervous, or reproductive systems. Adding to the confusion is the fact that the initial indications of many deficiencies are alarmingly similar: fatigue, weakness, minor aches and pains, headache, and so on.

Most researchers and practitioners in nutritional medicine agree, however, that certain physical clues point to specific nutrient deficiencies. For example, spoon-shaped fingernails with white spots, loss of the sense of smell or taste, and stretch marks are clinical signs of a zinc deficiency. These clues may be telling you that you are not taking in enough zinc, you have an increased need for the mineral, or you are not absorbing it.

Check Appendix B for a list of common physical symptoms and the associated nutrient deficiencies. While this list should not be used to try and make an exact diagnosis of your nutrient needs (other vitamins and minerals may also be involved), it gives the most common relationships and is a guide to help you establish which nutrients you may need to supplement. If some of the signs apply to you, circle the nutrients that correspond to the symptoms. Certain nutrients may appear more than once, indicating a likely deficiency. Before you run out and buy several bottles of vitamins, however, look at your diet. Are you eating foods that supply these nutrients? Are you engaging in habits that flush them out? Start here first to make needed changes.

Fine tuning your diet is a continuous exercise, because your needs vary day to day, month to month, and season to season. As we move to a new stage of development, or into unusual circumstances (having an operation, going on the Pill, fighting illness), we need to reevaluate and rebalance. What is correct for your body this month may not work in five years. Being tuned in to the workings of our bodies becomes a constant challenge and, as our bodies respond to our care and attention, a constant reward.

Your Plan of Action

+ Chart your dietary and lifestyle habits.

+ Check for nutrients taken in.

+ Check for nutrients depleted.

+ Determine your symptoms and signs.

+ Determine whether you have special needs (for example, high blood pressure).

+ Compare your diet to the proposed diet plan below.

EATING FOR LIFE

Use the following outline diet plan for comparison; it can help you to determine the areas in your diet that need improvement. Remember, it is a balanced food plan in itself, but it does not take into account special needs and biochemical differences.

Many women have no idea how many calories they should be eating in one day. There are many charts, and most of them conflict in the number and range of calories. I have found the following formula fairly accurate for a wide range of women. Keep in mind that it is an approximate number and is only a guide for redesigning your daily intake.

Proposed Diet Plan

LEVEL OF ACTIVITY	DAILY CALORIE INTAKE
Inactive women:	Ideal weight x 11
Moderately active women:	Ideal weight x 14
Active women:	Ideal weight x 18
Men:	Ideal weight x 18

Protein (12–15 percent of total diet)

Women:	40–60 g/day
Men:	45–75 g/day

FOOD	PROTEIN (GRAMS)

✦ Low fat (1 g or less)

Chicken breast, skinless (4 oz.)	35
Shellfish: shrimp, scallops, lobster (4 oz.)	23–35
Fish: cod, flounder, sole, halibut, trout (4 oz.)	21–30
Tuna, packed in water (2 oz.)	14
Cooked beans, peas, lentils (1 cup)	9–18
Tofu (4 oz.)	10
Milk, nonfat (1 cup)	8
Yogurt, nonfat (1 cup)	8
Pasta (1 cup)	7
Bulgur (1 cup)	6
Oatmeal (1 cup)	6
Macaroni (1 cup)	5
Bread, whole wheat (2 slices)	5
Rice, brown (1 cup)	5
Rice, white (1 cup)	4
Tortilla, flour (1 medium)	4

✦ Medium fat (1.5–3 g)

Beef, sirloin, choice or select (4 oz.)	34
Beef, bottom round, choice or select (4 oz.)	33
Chicken, dark meat (4 oz.)	29–31
Salmon (4 oz.)	31
Eggs (2, large)	13
Cheese, reduced fat (1 oz.)	8
Milk, 1 or 2 percent (1 cup)	8

✦ High fat (4–7 g)

Beef, chuck blade roast, choice or select (4 oz.)	35
Ground beef, regular, lean, or extra-lean (4 oz.)	28

FOOD	PROTEIN (GRAMS)
Mackerel (4 oz.)	28
Corned beef brisket (4 oz.)	21
Milk, whole (1 cup)	8
Peanut butter (2 Tbsps.)	8
Cheddar cheese (1 oz.)	7
Hot dog, beef or pork (2 oz.)	7

Carbohydrates (65–80 percent of total diet)

Increase complex carbohydrates (25–40 g/day of fiber)

Fruits (2–4 servings/day)

1 serving = 1 medium fruit, $\frac{1}{2}$ cup diced fruit, $\frac{3}{4}$ cup juice

Vegetables (4–5 servings/day)

1 serving = 1 cup raw or $\frac{1}{2}$ cup cooked

Breads, cereals, rice, pasta (6–11 servings/day)

1 serving = 1 slice bread; $\frac{1}{2}$ cup cooked cereal, pasta, or rice

Fats (20–25 percent of total diet)

Reduce saturated fats and trans fatty acids (red meats, butter, high-fat dairy, margarine, tropical oils, hydrogenated fats)

Increase monounsaturated oils (olive, canola, peanut)

Include essential fatty acids and omega-3 fatty acids (fish oils, salmon, trout, tuna, flaxseed oil)

18

DESIGNING YOUR
SUPPLEMENT PROGRAM

Preparing for menopause by eating the right foods and exercising is a great place to start, but it may not be enough to prevent menopausal symptoms or guard against bone loss. Women should consider the advantages of supplementation. The effectiveness of vitamin supplements and nutritional remedies in treating a variety of symptoms has been proven. Controlled scientific studies and epidemiological surveys have validated many of the theories of nutrition researchers in the last few years.

Providing the body with a complete supply of vitamins, minerals, enzymes, amino acids, fatty acids, trace elements, and fluids is the surest safeguard against poorly functioning glands, hormonal disturbances, and physiological imbalances. It is simple logic: when the restorative and regenerative cycles in the body are supplied with the raw materials they need, the body has a better chance to maintain optimum functioning.

One thing cannot be emphasized enough: supplements, even food-based vitamins and minerals, cannot replace healthful eating. Continuing to eat junk food while taking megadoses of vitamins is ridiculous—and probably dangerous. In fact, most supplements will not work in the context of an improper diet.

Supplements are best taken with food and with other nutrients. Vitamins and minerals rarely function independently. Whether any one nutrient is digested, absorbed, and properly utilized usually depends on the amount and availability of one or several others. If even one nutrient is missing, or in short supply, entire metabolic processes slow down or stop. Some of the interdependent nutrients you should remember from this book are calcium and magnesium, iron and vitamin C, and calcium and vitamin D.

How much of each vitamin and mineral do you personally need? No book can tell you this; it depends on your diet history, your family history, and clinical symptoms. The best that nutritionists and researchers can do is to provide guidelines and indicate the different nutrients that have benefited most individuals under specific, monitored circumstances. It is up to you to determine how closely your condition matches these standards, and to judge when you might need more or less, and when you need to revise your program. You know your body better than anyone else. Using the information in this book, you can analyze the data and work out your own program. If you are ever in doubt, or feel uneasy about the effects of your program, seek the guidance of a qualified nutritionist or consult your family doctor.

So, let us begin.

The nucleus of any supplement program is generally the multivitamin and mineral formula, and many women will find it meets most of their needs. Appendix A lists vitamins and minerals and the dosage ranges generally recommended by nutritionists and clinicians. Though some of the amounts go beyond RDA requirements, they are not unreasonable or excessive. When megadoses are called for, however, it is important to work with a physician; in large doses, any vitamin or mineral or other supplement acts as a drug and must be carefully monitored. If you have any doubts or questions about vitamin and mineral safety, I recommend consulting Patricia Hausman's The Right Dose.[1]

In addition to the basic formula outlined in Appendix A, further supplementation may be beneficial. If the multiple supplement you are taking doesn't contain an adequate amount of any nutrient (this is often true of calcium), or if you need a larger amount because of a specific problem (for example, vitamin E for breast pain), or if your daily habits are not going to change immediately (long-term smokers, drinkers, or coffee addicts), it would be wise to add single nutrients.

Supplement Safety

Supplement skeptics spend a good deal of time worrying about the alleged toxicity of vitamins and minerals. I think this needs to be addressed and put into perspective. According to the American Association of Poison Control Centers, the total number of accidental fatalities from legal FDA-approved prescription and over-the-counter drugs was 1,132 from 1983 to 1987. During this same time period, the total number of fatalities from vitamin supplements was zero. The incidence and likelihood of adverse reactions from supplement use are miniscule. The very few cases recorded in medical journals usually involved massive doses taken over long periods of time. That is not to say that overdose is impossible; it's just highly improbable. Extremely large doses of vitamins A and D can cause problems, but staying within the recommended doses is quite safe.

Natural Versus Synthetic

There is much confusion concerning the relative virtues of natural versus synthetic products. The naturalists claim that their products, derived chiefly from plant sources, contain still unidentified "associated cofactors"; for example, natural vitamin C contains the entire C complex, which makes it that much more effective, whereas synthetic C is just ascorbic acid, nothing more. Many clinicians I admire have found that natural vitamins are much less toxic when given in large amounts and they yield better results than the artificially produced varieties. On the other side of the debate are researchers with equally impressive degrees and experience. Those favoring synthetic products deny that there is any chemical difference, because in the test tube they all possess the same molecular properties. They also observe that, for people suffering from food allergies, the nonfood supplements are safer.

I don't predict any agreement between these two camps; however, there is a consensus on two nutrients: vitamin E and folic acid are better when taken from natural sources. Natural vitamin E (d-alpha tocopherol) is absorbed better than the synthetic (dl-alpha tocopherol). Don't be misled by labels that say the supplement contains vitamin E with d-alpha tocopherol; chances are the "with" greatly dilutes the active amount. As for folic acid, synthetic is the way to go, since it is more biologically available than the natural form.

Brand Name or Generic?

This issue is continually debated by the experts and manufacturers and, of course, they are not in agreement. The advice of Sheldon Hendler, author of *The Doctor's Vitamin and Mineral Encyclopedia*, is that all vitamins are essentially the same, so buy the least expensive.[2] "Only about a half-dozen drug companies actually make vitamins," say Hendler. They supply the basic raw materials, and the manufacturer mixes the blend, adding ingredients like sugar, coloring, bindings, and preservatives. However, many supplements list as many additives as they do nutrients, and personally, I think these should be avoided. When I hear that people have a difficult time digesting supplements, I often wonder if they might be allergic to one of the ingredients. If a supplement causes you distress, try another brand and see if it isn't better.

Dissolution Statement

Supplement manufacturers use a scientific procedure called a *disintegration test*, which mimics the action of the digestive tract, to test their products for dissolution and disintegration time. In January 1993, the US Pharmacopoeia (USP) adopted a voluntary supplement dissolution standard: water-soluble vitamins (B and C) should disintegrate in the digestive tract within 45 minutes. They expect to follow with a similar standard for fat-soluble vitamins. Look for information on the label about the supplier's testing procedures.

Expiration Dates

Not all supplements list a date, and even when they do, it does not guarantee freshness. Nevertheless, a date does suggest the manufacturer is aware that nutrients have a finite shelf life and is trying to offer a good product. If properly stored (covered, cool, and away from direct light), supplements retain their potency for two to three years from date of manufacturing. After opening, supplements keep up to one year.

Proceed Slowly

When you first begin your program, start slowly, adding one supplement at a time. If you have an allergic reaction to a particular ingredient, you will be able to determine the cause of the allergy more easily.

After a few months of a change in diet or supplementing, you should begin to notice subtle changes in your hair, eyes, fingernails, energy level, and sense of well-being. It is exciting to know that you can control to such a large extent how you feel and look by how well you nourish yourself and take care of your body.

Once you start your program to revamp your life and promote health and well-being, don't expect miracles. Nutrients don't work like drugs; they act slowly to rebuild tissue and reestablish homeostasis. If it has taken your body years to create a hormonal imbalance, don't expect it to reverse in a few days. It may actually take a few months. Be patient. Let the body mend in its own time. I must also mention that, as your body changes, you may actually feel worse for a few days before you feel better. This is normal, and you will find that the results are well worth the temporary transition.

The program you are designing now is not set in stone. Your needs, like your life, are constantly changing. Some changes are short-term (for example, pregnancy); others stay with us the rest of our lives. I continually readjust and fine tune my program as my lifestyle changes and my eating habits improve. And what I become more and more aware of is that the "purer" my daily intake—the less junk I put into my body—the less I need to supplement.

The real key to preparing for a healthy menopause—menopause without medicine—and a healthy second half of life is all-around good health: a nutritive diet, wise supplementation, regular physical exercise, and a positive mental attitude. Don't wait until you are going through the change to start thinking about your health. If you have prepared for the excitement and challenge of menopause far in advance of the midlife years, you will be ahead of the game, and your life will be the enjoyable, movable feast it was meant to be. Think about it, and start now.

Appendixes,
Glossary,
Chapter Notes,
Resources,
Index

APPENDIX A

A BASIC NUTRIENT
FORMULA FOR WOMEN

These dosages range from the RDA recommended amount to the higher therapeutic level. Some of the dosages recommended for the treatment of specific problems addressed in this book may exceed the amounts given below. Whenever using higher dosages, consult your health care professional.

NUTRIENTS	RANGE (RDA-THERAPEUTIC)†	TOXICITY LEVEL
Fat Soluble		
vitamin A (beta carotene)	5,000–20,000 IU or 15–30 mg	100,000 IU (retinol only)
vitamin D	400–800 IU	1,000 IU
vitamin E (d-alpha)	25–800 IU	3,000 IU
Water Soluble		
vitamin B-1 (thiamine)	1.4–100 mg	
vitamin B-2 (riboflavin)	1.2–100 mg	
vitamin B-3 (niacinamide)	19–100 mg	2,000 mg
vitamin B-6 (pyridoxine)	2–100 mg	200 mg
vitamin B-12 (cobalamine)	2–200 mcg	
vitamin C	60–5,000 mg	

NUTRIENTS	RANGE (RDA-THERAPEUTIC)†	TOXICITY LEVEL
vitamin K	70–500 mcg	
bioflavenoids	500–2,000 mg	
biotin*	150–300 mcg	
choline*	50–100 mg	
folic acid	200–800 mcg	
inositol*	50–100 mg	
lecithin		
pantothenic acid*	7–200 mg	
Minerals		
boron	3 mg	
calcium	800–2,000 mg	3,000 mg
chromium*	200–600 mcg	
copper*	2–3 mg	
iodine (kelp)	150 mcg	1,000 mcg
iron	18–30 mg	100 mg
magnesium	300–800 mg	8,000 mg
manganese*	2.5–10 mg	
potassium*	1,875–5,625 mg	
selenium	70–400 mcg	1,000 mcg
sodium*	1,100–3,300 mg	
zinc	15–50 mg	2,000 mg

* No RDA established.

† Individual chapter recommendations may be specific to a symptom or problem. The ranges given here are general to therapeutic.

APPENDIX B

CLINICAL SYMPTOMS OF NUTRIENT DEFICIENCIES

Ca—calcium
Cr—chromium
Cu—copper
EFA—essential fatty acids
Fe—iron
I—iodine

K—potassium
Mg—Magnesium
PABA—para-aminobenzoic acid
Se—selenium
Zn—zinc

BODY AREA	SYMPTOM	POSSIBLE DEFICIENCY
Skin	dry, flaky	A, B, E, EFA
	oily	B-complex (especially B-6, choline, inositol)
	bruise easily	C, K
	wounds heal slowly	C, Zn
	yellow color	B-6, choline, Mg
	brown pigmentation	B, C, E
	prominent veins	C, bioflanvenoids, Zn
	pale, white	B, C, Fe
	stretch marks on hips, thighs, breasts	B, E, Zn
	backs of arms rough	A
Nails	brittle	Fe, Ca, protein, EFA
	white spots	Zn, Ca
	spoon-shaped	Fe, Zn
Eyes	dark circles underneath	B, K
	small yellow lumps on white part	A, E, Zn
	night blindness, dry eyes	A

BODY AREA	SYMPTOM	POSSIBLE DEFICIENCY
	red blood vessels around corners	general poor health
Hair	dull, dry	protein
	oily	choline, inositol
	hair splits and grows poorly	protein, Zn
	dermatitis	B, Zn, EFA
	hair thins out	B, protein, EFA
	dandruff	B
Mouth	canker sores	A, B-complex, Zn
	bad breath	B-complex (especially B-3)
	cracks on corner of lips	B-1, B-2, B-3
Tongue	magenta coating	B-complex (especially B-12), K
	green cast	B-complex (especially B-6, choline)
	white	B-complex (especially choline), C
	thick white spots	A, B-complex
	scalloped sides	B-6, B-12, folic acid
Teeth and gums	bleeding and spongy gums	C, B-complex
	cavities	B-complex, Ca, Zn
	grinding teeth	Ca, Mg
	periodontal disease	Ca
Gastro-intestinal system	enlarged liver	B-complex (especially choline, inositol), protein, lecithin
	nausea	A, B-3, B-6, Mg
	hemorrhoids	B-6, C, bioflavenoids, Mg
	bloating (gas)	B-complex, Zn
	hard bowel movement (infrequent)	Fe, fiber
Respiratory system	prone to infections	A, B-complex, C
	sinus	A, B-complex, C, K, Zn
	loss of sense of smell	A, B-complex, Zn

BODY AREA	SYMPTOM	POSSIBLE DEFICIENCY
	dry membranes	A, D, E, Zn
Cardiovascular system	increased heart rate	B-complex, C, E, Ca, Mg
	slow, irregular heartbeat	B-complex, K
	elevated blood pressure	Choline, Ca, K, Se, Cr
Muscular/ skeletal	muscle weakness	B-complex, K
	muscle cramps	D, B-5, Ca, Mg
	stiff joints	B-complex, Ca, Mg
General	cold hands and feet	I
	loss of sense of taste	Zn
	insomnia	D, Ca, Mg
	varicose veins	C, E, Fe, Cu
	nervousness	B-complex (especially PABA), Ca, Mg
	low energy	B-complex, I, Fe
	poor memory	B-complex (especially inositol, choline), I, Mg
	inability to recall dreams	B-6
	frequent ear wax	B-complex (especially choline, inositol),

Sources: Jeffrey Bland, Ph.D., *Nutraerobics* (New York: Harper and Row, 1983); Richard A. Kunin, M.D., *Mega-Nutrition for Women* (New York: McGraw-Hill, 1983).

APPENDIX C

Major Nutrient Guide

VITAMIN A

beef liver (3 oz.)	45,400 IU
carrot (1, medium)	7,900
sweet potato, cooked (½ cup)	7,850
pumpkin, cooked (½ cup)	7,840
spinach, cooked (½ cup)	7,300
cantaloupe (½)	5,400
tomato juice (¾ cup)	1,460

Other sources: squash, red peppers, eggs, peaches, Swiss chard, endive, beet greens, broccoli, papaya, crab
Depleters: ERT, heat, coffee, processed foods, low-fat diet

VITAMIN B-1: THIAMINE

brewer's yeast (2 Tbsps.)	3.00 mg
sunflower seeds (1 cup)	2.84
split peas, cooked (1 cup)	1.48
black beans (1 cup)	1.10
pecans (1 cup)	0.96
wheat germ, toasted (¼ cup)	0.44
asparagus (1 cup)	0.24

Other sources: oatmeal, peanuts, liver, brown rice, fish
Depleters: heat, ERT, stress, sulfa drugs, sugar, processed foods, cigarettes, alcohol, dieting, surgery, illness, coffee, tea

VITAMIN B-2: RIBOFLAVIN

beef liver (3 oz.)	3.65 mg
brussels sprouts (1 cup)	2.00
almonds (1 cup)	1.31
brewer's yeast (3 Tbsps.)	1.00
split peas, cooked (1 cup)	0.58
milk (1 cup)	0.34

broccoli, cooked (1 cup)   0.31

Other sources: organ meats, wheat cereals, burritos, red meats, yogurt, eggs, poultry, wheat germ, nuts, sesame seeds

Depleters: alcohol, antibiotics, ERT, light, stress, junk foods, sulfa drugs, coffee, tea

VITAMIN B-3: NIACIN/NIACINAMIDE

tuna, in water (1 cup)	47.3 mg
chicken, light meat (3 oz.)	10.0
broccoli (1 cup)	9.7
sunflower seeds (1 cup)	9.0
mushrooms (1 cup)	5.7
haddock (6 oz.)	5.4
peanut butter (21 Tbsps.)	2.4

Other sources: pumpkin and squash seeds, cashews, uncreamed cottage cheese, split peas, beans, avocado, brewer's yeast

Depleters: sugar, antibiotics, alcohol, coffee, stress, ERT, sulfa drugs, sleeping pills

VITAMIN B-6: PYRIDOXINE

brown rice (1 cup)	1.00 mg
tuna, in water (1 cup)	0.85
beef liver (3 oz.)	0.84
chicken, white meat (3 oz.)	0.68
banana (1, medium)	0.76
fresh chestnuts, (1 cup)	0.53

Other sources: sunflower seeds, alfalfa sprouts, wheat germ, fish, prunes, avocado, cabbage, grapes, green peas

Depleters: ERT, cortisone, penicillin, heat, light, high protein diet, sugar, alcohol, stress, coffee

VITAMIN C

kiwi fruit (1)	108 mg
orange juice (6 oz.)	87
orange (1)	85
broccoli, cooked (½ cup)	70
brussels sprouts, cooked (½ cup)	65
grapefruit juice (6 oz.)	57
strawberries (½ cup)	48
tomato, raw (1)	46
potato (1)	29

Other sources: raw green peppers, cantaloupe, grapes, watermelon

Depleters: stress, cigarettes, pollution

VITAMIN D

canned tuna/salmon (1/4 lb.)	400 IU
whole milk (1 cup)	100
beef liver (1/4 lb.)	40
butter (1 oz.)	28
egg yolk (1)	27

Other sources: fatty fish, organ meats, shrimp, fish liver oils, sun
Depleters: smog, mineral oil, cortisone, anticonvulsants

VITAMIN E

sunflower seeds (1/4 cup)	27.1 IU
raw filberts (1 cup)	13.5
almonds (1 cup)	12.7
cucumber, raw (1 cup)	12.6
kale, raw (1 cup)	12.0
coleslaw (1 cup)	10.5
crab (6 oz.)	9.0

Other sources: vegetable oils, asparagus, whole-wheat breads, eggs, liver, collards, peanuts, wheat germ
Depleters: ERT, mineral oil, chlorine, freezing, heat, oxygen, thyroid hormone, excess polyunsaturated oil

VITAMIN K

broccoli (1/2 cup)	168 mg
lettuce (1/2 cup)	108
cabbage (1/2 cup)	105
spinach (1/2 cup)	75
asparagus (1/2 cup)	48

Depleters: It is not known what depletes vitamin K.

FOLIC ACID

brewer's yeast (1 Tbsp.)	313 mcg
black-eyed peas (1/2 cup)	230
orange juice (1 cup)	136
beef liver (3 oz.)	123
romaine lettuce (1 cup)	98
cantaloupe (1/2)	82

Other sources: spinach, broccoli, beets, brussels sprouts, potatoes, almonds
Depleters: alcohol, stress, ERT, heat, light, oxygen, sulfa drugs, sugar, caffeine

CALCIUM

sardines (4 oz.)	496 mg
almonds (1 cup)	333
whole milk (1 cup)	298
yogurt, skim milk (1 cup)	294
salmon, with bones (3 oz.)	275
tofu (4 oz.)	154
broccoli (1 cup)	136

Other sources: cheese, corn tortillas, pinto beans, blackstrap molasses, sunflower seeds, chick-peas, kale

Depleters: antibiotics, cigarettes, high protein diets, sugar, fat, oxalic acid in spinach, inactivity

IRON

beef liver (3 oz.)	7.5 mg
wheat bran (½ cup)	7.2
pistachios (1 cup)	7.2
sunflower seeds (½ cup)	5.1
dried apricots (½ cup)	3.6
blackstrap molasses (1 Tbsp.)	3.2
almonds (½ cup)	2.7
raisins (½ cup)	2.5
tofu (4 oz.)	2.5

Other sources: turkey, haddock, spinach, pumpkin seeds, cashews, lima beans, soybeans, peanuts, sprouts, peas, brewer's yeast

Depleters: ERT, blood loss, high altitude, coffee, tea

MAGNESIUM

peanuts (¼ cup)	247 mg
lentils, cooked (½ cup)	134
tofu (4 oz.)	126
wheat germ (¼ cup)	97
almonds (¼ cup)	96
shredded wheat (1 cup)	67
banana (1, medium)	58
oatmeal (1 cup)	50

Other sources: split peas, kidney beans, potatoes, raw spinach, brown rice, salmon, milk, most nuts

Depleters: diuretics, alcohol, ERT, phytic acid in whole grains, large amounts of zinc or fluoride

beef liver (3 oz.)	7.7 mg
mushrooms (1 cup)	2.7
sunflower seeds (1 cup)	2.0
wheat bran (1 cup)	1.6
egg (1)	1.6
cabbage, raw (1 cup)	1.3

Other sources: cashews, whole grains, wheat germ, salmon, beans, broccoli, peas, avocado, milk, chicken, peanut butter, bananas, potatoes

Depleters: heat, stress, methyl bromide, alcohol, sugar, coffee, cigarettes

POTASSIUM

fish (6 oz.)	760 mg
papaya (1 medium)	710
cantaloupe (½)	682
butternut squash, cooked (½ cup)	600
lima beans (½ cup)	600
blackstrap molasses (1 Tbsp.)	585
prunes (½ cup)	559
orange juice (1 cup)	496

Other sources: spinach, pinto beans, halibut, banana, potato, sweet potato, green pepper, peach, apricot, tomato, soybeans, watermelon

Depleters: diuretics, laxatives, malnutrition, fasting, surgery, ERT, sugar, stress, coffee, alcohol

SELENIUM

lobster (6 oz.)	132 mcg
tuna (6 oz.)	120
shrimp (6 oz.)	108
ham (6 oz.)	58
egg (1)	37

Other sources: chicken, whole-wheat breads, whole grain cereals

Depleters: It is not known what depletes selenium. Some parts of the country have selenium-depleted soils; produce from those areas will not have the selenium content of produce from other areas.

ZINC

Pacific oysters (100 g)	9.0 mg
Brazil nuts, raw (1 cup)	7.1
cashews (1 cup)	6.1
turkey, dark meat (3 oz.)	4.0
turkey, light meat (3 oz.)	2.0
white fish (6 oz.)	2.0
wheat germ (1 Tbsp.)	1.0

Other sources: red meat, almonds, lobster, whole grains, eggs, bran flakes, lentils, soybean sprouts

Depleters: infection, pernicious anemia, overactive thyroid, excess sweating, alcohol, diabetes, large amounts of vitamins B and C

APPENDIX D

STRENGTHENING EXERCISES FOR WOMEN

The muscle strengthening exercises presented here have been specially designed to be of maximum benefit for menopausal women. Before you begin any exercise regimen, see your doctor for a complete physical, and review the exercises with him or her. If specific exercises, or a high level of exertion, are contraindicated, do not proceed except under supervision. Always stop if you experience ongoing pain or joint soreness. Remember, no amount of exercise is healthful if it is harming any part of your body.

The exercises are illustrated in two positions: A, the starting position, and B, the finishing position. Read the complete exercise before attempting it. Pay particular attention to the "don'ts" that are shown by the figures in the illustrations.

Repetitions for all dumbbell movements: Two sets of 15 repetitions for five-pound weights. Fewer repetitions are required for heavier weights, more for lighter.

Cautions for all standing exercises: Keep back straight and knees slightly bent. Hold stomach muscles in. Keep breathing and control the movement.

Cautions for floor stomach exercises: Do not arch your back. Check with your hand to make sure your lower back touches the floor. Pull up with your stomach muscles and not with your neck. Control the movement at all times.

Exercise 1—Alternate Dumbbell Curl

Benefit: Tones the biceps and forearms.

Stand with torso straight and knees slightly bent. Hold a dumbbell in each hand with arms bent at the waist and palms facing upward. Keeping elbows close to the sides, raise one weight while the other arm remains bent at the waist. Repeat this motion with the other arm and continue to alternate. Repeat 12 times for each arm, then rest and repeat 12 more times.

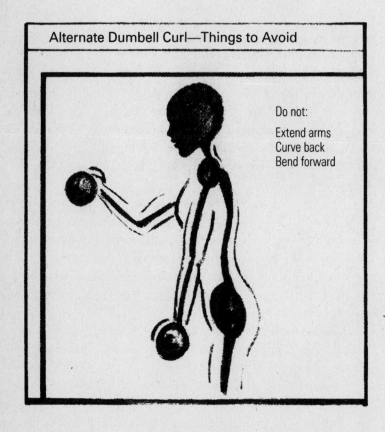

Alternate Dumbell Curl—Things to Avoid

Do not:

Extend arms
Curve back
Bend forward

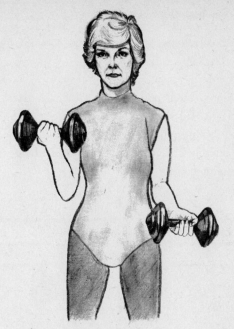

A

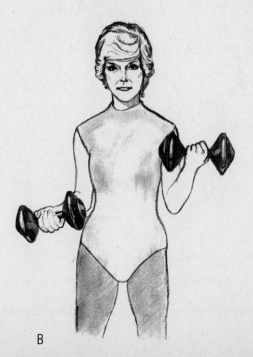

B

Exercise 2—Dumbbell Press

Benefit: Works all three sections of the shoulder muscles (deltoids), triceps, and upper chest.

Stand or sit erect. Hold one dumbbell in each hand at shoulder level. Weights should be parallel to the floor and palms facing forward. Press dumbbell slowly overhead as you exhale. Inhale and slowly lower dumbbell back to shoulder level. Repetitions are the same as for Exercise 1.

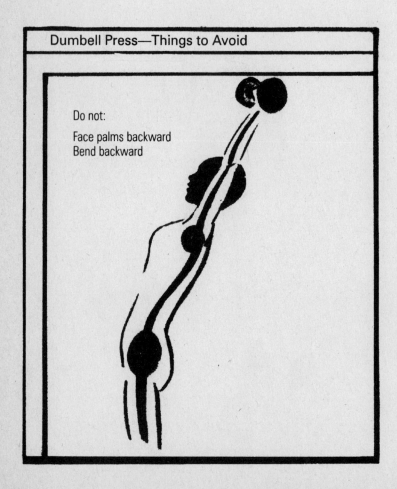

Dumbell Press—Things to Avoid

Do not:

Face palms backward
Bend backward

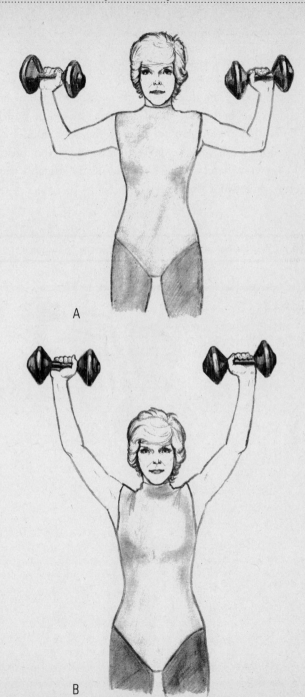

A

B

Exercise 3—Two-Arm Dumbbell Extension

Benefit: An all-around triceps developer.

Stand or sit, clasping one dumbbell with both hands, palms facing upward. Raise dumbbell above the head. Arms should be pulled all the way up so that the elbows are close to the ears. Inhale as you lower the dumbbell behind your head. Exhale as you raise the dumbbell over your head until elbows are nearly straight. Repetitions are the same as for Exercise 1.

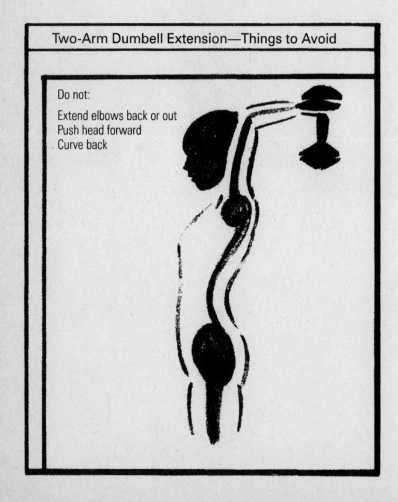

Two-Arm Dumbell Extension—Things to Avoid

Do not:

Extend elbows back or out
Push head forward
Curve back

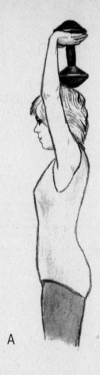

A

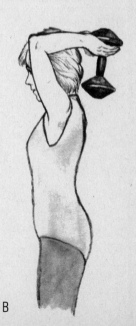

B

Exercise 4—Arm Pull

Benefit An all-around shoulder and arm developer.

Stand with knees and waist slightly bent, stomach and buttock muscles held firm. Hold arms directly in front of you. Pull back to the waist and then push arms straight. Extend and pull as many times as you can until your arms get tired. Wearing or holding weights makes the exercise more effective.

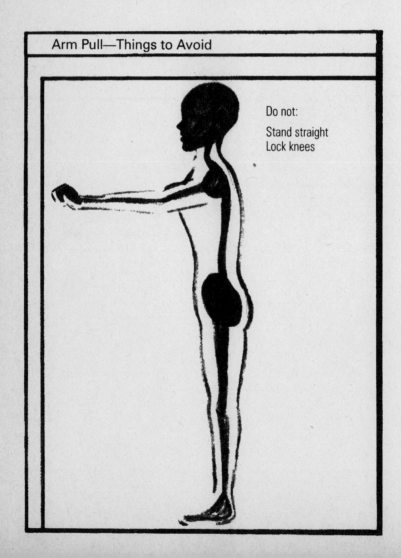

Arm Pull—Things to Avoid

Do not:

Stand straight
Lock knees

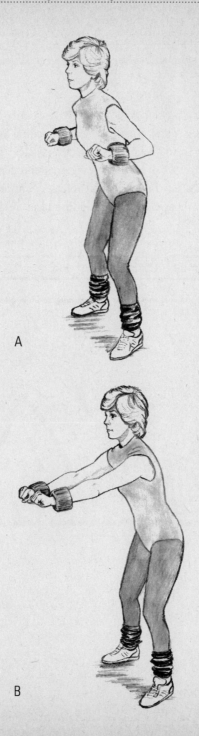

A

B

Exercise 5—Sit-up Crunch

Benefit: Strengthens abdominal muscles directly and back muscles indirectly.

Lie on the floor on your back, with knees bent. With arms extended above chest, point hands toward the ceiling and look directly up. Raise upper torso, keeping stomach muscles tight and lower back pressed to the floor at all times. Be careful not to arch back. Exhale as you curl up, inhale as you release. Stay in control at all times. Go for 20 repetitions to start and add more as you are able.

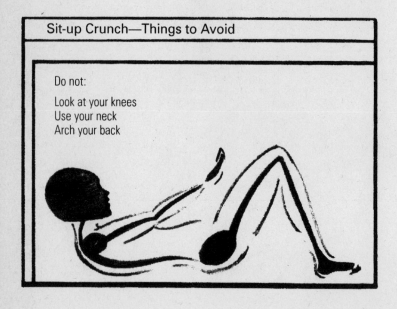

Sit-up Crunch—Things to Avoid

Do not:

Look at your knees
Use your neck
Arch your back

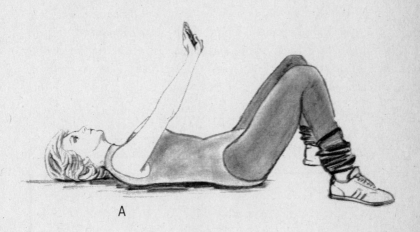

A

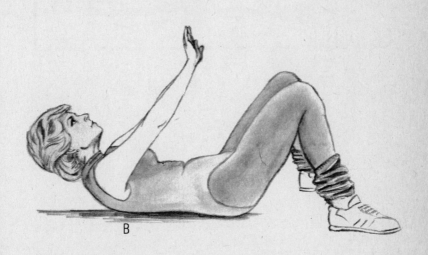

B

Exercise 6—Side Sit-Up

Benefit: Strengthens the obliques (side stomach muscles).

Lie on the floor on back, with legs bent and dropped to one side. Fold arms and place them behind the head to support neck. Looking up at the ceiling, exhale and lift up. Inhale as you lower both legs to the other side. Start with 20 repetitions, and work up to 50 on each side.

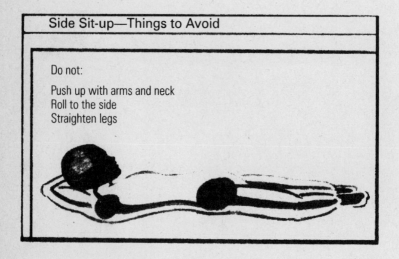

Side Sit-up—Things to Avoid

Do not:

Push up with arms and neck
Roll to the side
Straighten legs

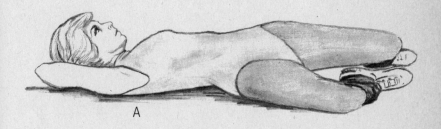

A

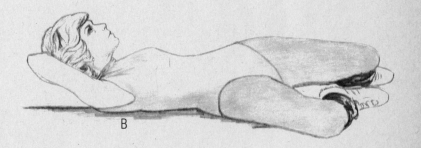

B

Exercise 7—Bicycle Twist

Benefit: Works the stomach, waist, shoulders, and upper thighs.

Lie on the floor on your back, with arms clasped behind the head and legs straight. Lift both the left shoulder and the right knee off the floor simultaneously. Bring them as close together as is comfortably possible—without pulling on your neck. Reverse arm and leg and continue cycling motion until tired.

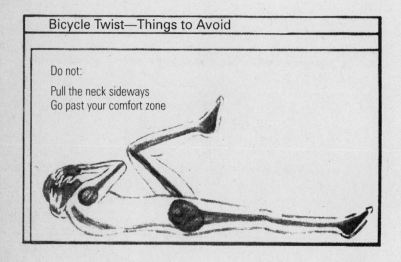

Bicycle Twist—Things to Avoid

Do not:

Pull the neck sideways
Go past your comfort zone

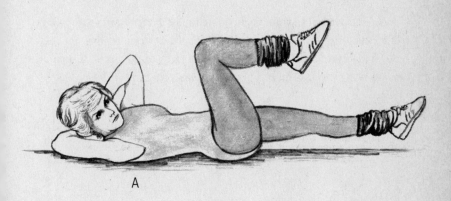

A

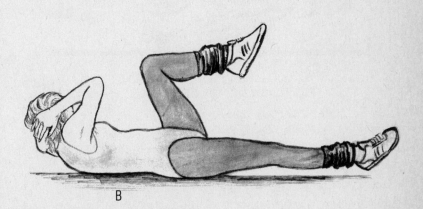

B

Exercise 8—Pelvic Tilt

Benefit: Strengthens and tones the stomach, buttocks, lower back, and internal organs. Also reverses the flow of blood and stimulates circulation.

Lie on the floor on your back, with knees bent. Raise the lower trunk, keeping upper back on the floor. Raise four to five inches, hold, and then lower. Keep the buttocks tight at all times. Remember, do not raise too high. Do as many as you can.

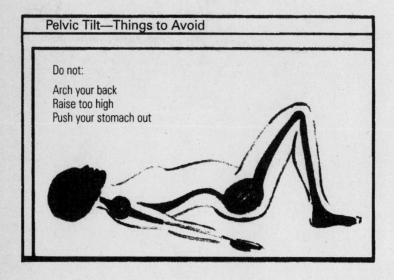

Pelvic Tilt—Things to Avoid

Do not:

Arch your back
Raise too high
Push your stomach out

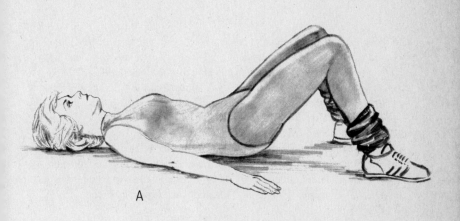

A

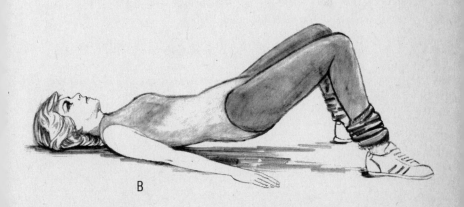

B

Chapter Notes

Chapter 1

1. Robert A. Wilson, *Feminine Forever* (New York: M. Evans, 1966).
2. David R. Reuben, M.D., *Everything You Always Wanted to Know about Sex, but Were Afraid to Ask* (New York: Hawthorne Books, 1977), 292.
3. N. E. Avis and S. M. McKinlay, "A Longitudinal Analysis of Women's Attitudes Toward the Menopause: Results from the Massachusetts Women's Health Study," *Maturitas* 13 (1991): 65–79.
4. Sheldon H. Cherry, M.D., *For Women of All Ages: A Gynecologist's Guide to Modern Female Health Care* (New York: Macmillan, 1979), 205.
5. M. C. Martin, J. E. Block, S. D. Sanchez, et al., "Menopause Without Symptoms: The Endocrinology of Menopause Among Rural Mayan Indians," *American Journal of Obstetrics and Gynecology* 168 (1993): 1839–45.
6. Cathy Perlmutter, Toby Hanlon, and Maureen Sangiorgio, "Triumph over Menopause: Results from Our Exclusive Woman-to-Woman Survey with the Center for Women's Health at Columbia-Presbyterian Medical Center, New York," *Prevention* (August 1994).
7. Cherry, *For Women of All Ages*, 205.
8. Barbara Evans, M.D., *Life Change: A Guide to the Menopause, Its Effects and Treatment* (London: Pan Books, 1979), 92.
9. Kaylan Pickford, *Always a Woman* (New York: Bantam Books, 1982).
10. Howard J. Osofsky, M.D., and Robert Seidenburg, M.D., "Is Female Menopausal Depression Inevitable?" *Obstetrics/Gynecology* 36 (October 1970): 611–14.
11. Juanita Williams, *Psychology of Women* (New York: W. W. Norton, 1977), 360.
12. Maxwell Maltz, *Psycho-Cybernetics* (Englewood Cliffs NJ: Prentice-Hall, 1960).

Chapter 2

1. R. J. Beard, ed., *The Menopause: A Guide to Current Research and Practice* (Lancaster, England: MTP Press, 1976), 30; Edmund R. Novak, M.D., Robert B. Greenblatt, M.D., and Herbert S. Kupperman, M.D., "Treating Menopausal Women—and Climacteric Men," *Medical World News* (July 28, 1974): 32–44.
2. Beard, *The Menopause*, 27.
3. Hershel Jick, Jane Porter, and Alan S. Morrison, "Relation Between Smoking and Age of Natural Menopause" (Report from the Boston Collaborative Drug Surveillance Program, Boston University Medical

Center), *Lancet* 1 (June 25, 1977): 1354–55.

4. Louisa Rose, ed., *The Menopause Book* (New York: Hawthorne Books, Inc., 1977), 22.

5. Lila Nachtigall, M.D., with Joan Heilman, *The Lila Nachtigall Report* (New York: G. P. Putnam, 1977), 165.

6. Barbara Evans, M.D., *Life Change: A Guide to the Menopause, Its Effects and Treatment* (London: Pan Books, 1979), 92.

7. Rosetta Reitz, *Menopause: A Positive Approach* (Radnor PA: Chilton, 1977), 19.

8. Louis Parish, M.D., *No Pause at All* (New York: Readers Digest Press, 1977), 30.

9. Winnifred Berg Cutler, Ph.D., Celso-Ramon Garcia, M.D., and David A. Edwards, Ph.D., *Menopause: A Guide for Women and the Men Who Love Them* (New York: W. W. Norton, 1983), 66.

10. Penny Wise Budoff, M.D., *No More Hot Flashes and Other Good News* (New York: G. P. Putnam, 1983), 19.

11. Beard, *The Menopause*, 46.

12. Howard L. Judd, M.D., "Menopause and Postmenopause," in Ralph C. Benson, M.D., *Current Obstetric and Gynecologic Diagnosis and Treatment*, 4th ed. (Los Altos CA: Lange Medical Publications, 1982), 550.

13. Barbara Seaman and Gideon Seaman, M.D., *Women and the Crisis in Sex Hormones* (New York: Bantam Books, 1979), 365.

Chapter 3

1. Margaret Locke, "Contested Meanings of the Menopause," *Lancet* 337 (1991): 1270–72.

2. Martin, Block, Sanchez, et al., "Menopause Without Symptoms: The Endocrinology of Menopause among Rural Mayan Indians," *American Journal Obstetrics and Gynecology* 168 (1993): 1839–45.

3. H. Aldercreutz, E. Hamalainen, S. Gorbach, and B. Goldin, "Dietary Phyto-oestrogens and the Menopause in Japan, *Lancet* 339 (1992): 1233.

4. Niels H. Lauersen, M.D., and Eileen Stukane, *Listen to Your Body: A Gynecologist Answers Women's Most Intimate Questions* (New York: Berkley Books, 1983), 377.

5. Mats Hammar, Goran Berg, and Richard Lindgren, "Does Physical Exercise Influence the Frequency of Postmenopausal Hot Flashes?" *Acta Obstet Gynecol Scand* 69 (1990): 409–12.

6. Robert Freedman and Suzanne Woodward, "Behavioral Treatment of Menopausal Hot Flushes: Evaluation by Ambulatory Monitoring," *American Journal of Obstetrics and Gynecology* 167 (1992): 436–39.

7. John Yudkin, M.D., *Sweet and Dangerous* (New York: Bantam Books, 1973), 164.

8. Federation of Feminist Women's Health Centers, *A New View of a Woman's Body* (New York: Simon and Schuster, 1981), 96.

9. G. Wilcox, M. L. Wahlqvist, H. G. Burger, and G. Medley, "Oestrogenic Effects of Plant Foods in Postmenopausal Women," *British Medical Journal* 301 (1990): 905–6.

10. Mark Messina and Stephan Barnes, "Commentary: The Role of Soy Products in Reducing the Risk of Cancer," *Journal of the National Cancer Institute* 83 (1991): 541–46.

11. H. Aldercreutz, H. Markkanen, and S. Watanabe, "Plasma Concentration of Phyto-oestrogens in Japanese Men," *Lancet* 342 (1993): 1209–10.

12. J. T. Dwyer, B. R. Goldin, N. Saul, et al., "Tofu and Soy Drinks Contain Phytoestrogens," *Journal of the American Dietetic Association* 94 (1994): 739–43.

13. Rami Kaldas and Hugh Claud, "Reproductive and General Metabolic Effects of Phytoestrogen in Mammals," *Reproductive Toxicology* Vol 3 No 2 (1989): 81–89.

14. G. J. Christy, "Vitamin E in Menopause: Preliminary Reports of Experimental and Clinical Study," American *Journal of Obstetrics and Gynecology* 50 (1945): 84.

15. Michael Lesser, M.D., *Nutrition and Vitamin Therapy* (New York: Grove Press, 1980), 98.

16. Barbara Seaman and Gideon Seaman, M.D., *Women and the Crisis in Sex Hormones* (New York: Bantam Books, 1979), 445.

17. Sarah Harriman, *The Book of Ginseng* (New York: Jove, 1973), 25.

18. Robert C. Atkins, *Dr. Atkins' Nutrition Breakthrough: How to Treat Your Medical Condition Without Drugs* (New York: William Morrow, 1981), 131.

Chapter 4

1. Barbara Edelstein, M.D., *The Woman Doctor's Medical Guide for Women* (New York: William Morrow, 1982), 82.

2. William Dufty, *Sugar Blues* (New York: Warner Books, 1975), 43.

3. R. O. Brennan, M.D., with William C. Mulligan, *Nutrigenetics: New Concepts for Relieving Hypoglycemia* (New York: Signet Books, 1977), 9.

4. Clement G. Martin, M.D., *Low Blood Sugar: The Hidden Menace of Hypoglycemia* (New York: Arco Publishing, 1981), 41.

5. Earl Mindell, *Earl Mindell's Vitamin Bible* (New York: Rawson, Wade, 1979), 176.

6. G. Collier and K. O'Dea, "Effect of Physical Form of Carbohydrate on the Postprandial Glucose, Insulin, and Gastric Inhibitory Polypeptide in Type 2 Diabetes," *American Journal of Clinical Nutrition* 36 (1982): 10.

7. T. Poynard and G. Tchobroutsky, "Pectin Efficacy in Insulin-Treated Diabetes," *Lancet* (January 18, 1980): 158.

8. Jeffrey Bland and Scott Rigden, A *Physician and Patient Survival Guide: Resource Guide Treating the Burnout Syndrome* (Gig Harbor WA: Health Communication, 1987), 87.

9. R. A. Anderson, M. Polansky, N. Bryden, et al., "Urinary Chromium Excretion of Human Subjects: Effects of Chromium Supplementation

and Glucose Loading," *American Journal of Clinical Nutrition* 36 (1982): 118–24.

10. Julian Whitaker, M.D., "99 Medical Secrets Your Doctor Won't Tell You," *Health and Healing,* (Potomac MD: Phillips Publishing, 1993).

11. Brennan, *Nutrigenetics,* 160.

12. Richard A. Kunin, M.D., *Mega-Nutrition* (New York: McGraw-Hill, 1981), 125.

13. Broda Barnes, M.D., and Charlotte Barnes, *Hope for Hypoglycemia* (Fort Collins CO: Robinson Press, 1978), 11.

14. Kunin, *Mega-Nutrition,* 86.

15. "Essential Trace Elements and Thyroid Hormones," *Lancet* 339 (1992): 1575–76.

16. Georgia Witkin-Lanoil, Ph.D., *The Female Stress Syndrome: How to Recognize and Live with It* (New York: Newmarket Press, 1984).

17. J. Kleijnen and P. Knipschild, "Drug Profiles—Ginko Biloba," *Lancet* 340 (1993): 1136–39.

Chapter 5

1. Shere Hite, *The Hite Report: A Nationwide Study of Female Sexuality* (New York: Dell, 1981), 508.

2. Linda Madaras, Jane Patterson, and Peter Schlick, *Womancare: Gynecological Guide to Your Body* (New York: Avon, 1981), 611.

3. Norma McCoy, Winnifred Cutler, and Julian Davidson, "Relationships among Sexual Behavior, Hot Flashes, and Hormone Levels in Perimenopausal Women," *Archives of Sexual Behavior* 14 (1985): 385–88.

4. Lauersen and Stukane, *Listen to Your Body,* 386.

5. H. Adlercreutz, H. Honjo, A. Higashi, et al., "Urinary Excretion of Lignans and Isoflavenoids, Phytoestrogens in Japanese Men and Women Consuming a Traditional Japanese Diet," *American Journal of Clinical Nutrition* 54 (1991): 1093–1100.

6. Dwyer, Goldin, Saul, et al., "Tofu and Soy Drinks" 739–743.

7. John Lee, M.D., *Natural Progesterone: The Multiple Roles of a Remarkable Hormone,* (Sebastopol CA: BLL Publishing, 1993), 58.

8. J. Ofek, J. Goldhar, D. Zafriri, et al., "Anti-Escherichia Coli Adhesion Activity of Cranberry and Blueberry Juice," *New England Journal of Medicine* 324 (1991): 1599.

9. Vidal S. Clay, *Women: Menopause and Middle Age* (Pittsburgh PA: Know, 1977), 92.

10. Jeffrey Bland, Ph.D., *Nutraerobics,* (New York: Harper and Row, 1983), 17.

11. Durk Pearson and Sandy Shaw, *Life Extension: A Practical Scientific Approach* (New York: Warner Books, 1982), 205.

Chapter 6

1. J. B. McKinlay, S. M. McKinlay, and D. Bramvilla, "The Relative

Contributions of Endocrine Changes and Social Circumstances to Depression in Middle-Aged Women," *Journal of Health and Social Behavior* 28 (1987): 345–63.

2. Sadja Greenwood, M.D., *Menopause Naturally: Preparing for the Second Half of Life* (San Francisco: Volcano Press, 1984), 73.

3. Lonnie Barbach, Ph.D., *The Pause: Positive Approaches to Menopause* (New York: Penguin Books, 1993), 41.

4. Barbara Edelstein, M.D., *The Woman Doctor's Medical Guide for Women* (New York: William Morrow, 1982), 132.

5. Margaret Lock, "Contested Meanings of Menopause," *Lancet* 337 (1991): 1270–72.

6. Allan Chinen, M.D., *Once upon a Midlife* (New York: Jeremy P. Tarcher/Perigee, 1993), 211.

7. William Bridges, *Transitions* (Reading MA: Addison-Wesley Publishing Company, 1980), 14.

8. Gloria Steinem, *Revolution from Within: A Book of Self-Esteem* (Boston: Little, Brown and Company, 1992), 3.

9. Lillian B. Rubin, *Women of a Certain Age: The Midlife Search for Self* (New York: Harper and Row, 1979), 54.

10. Pauline Bart, "Depression in Middle-Aged Women," in Vivian Gornick and Barbara K. Moran, eds., *Woman in Sexist Society: Studies in Power and Powerlessness* (New York: Basic Books, 1971), 110.

11. Judith Wurtman, *Managing Your Mind and Mood Through Food* (New York: Harper and Row, 1988), 5.

12. Debra Waterhouse, "The Brain-Body Connection: Hormones, Diet and Behavior," seminar, Corte Madera, CA: Institute for Natural Resources, 1993.

13. Mona M. Shangold, "Exercise in the Menopausal Woman," *Obstetrics and Gynecology* 75 (1990): 53S.

14. *American Health* (March/April 1984): 28.

15. E. Cheraskin, M.D., and W. M. Ringdorf, Jr., with Arline Brecher, *Psychodietetics: Food as Key to Emotional Health* (New York: Bantam Books, 1981), 72.

16. Roger J. Williams, Ph.D., *Nutrition in a Nutshell* (Garden City NY: Doubleday, 1962), 94.

17. Jos Kleijnen and Paul Knipschild, "Ginko Biloba," *Lancet* 340 (1993): 1136–39.

Chapter 7

1. Lois McBean, Tab Forgac, and Susan Calvert Finn, "Osteoporosis: Visions for Care and Prevention—A Conference Report," *Journal of the American Diabetic Association* 94 (1994): 668–71.

2. Morris Notelovitz, M.D., and Marsha Ware, *Stand Tall! The Informed Woman's Guide to Preventing Osteoporosis* (Gainesville, FL: Triad Publishing, 1982), 40.

3. Howard L. Judd, M.D., "Menopause and Postmenopause," in Ralph C. Benson, M.D., *Current Obstetric and Gynecologic Diagnosis and Treatment*, 4th ed. (Los Altos CA: Lange Medical Publications, 1982), 554.

4. Thomas J. Silber, "Osteoporosis in Anorexia Nervosa," *New England Journal of Medicine* 312 (1985): 990–91.

5. *American Journal of Clinical Nutrition* (June 1986): 910.

6. C. Rosen, M. Holick, and P. Millard, "Premature Graying of Hair Is a Risk Maker for Osteopenia," *Journal of Clinical Endocrinology and Metabolism* 79 (1994): 854–57.

7. Notelovitz and Ware, *Stand Tall!* 72.

8. Bland, *Nutraerobics*, 256.

9. N. A. Breslau, L. Brinkley, K. D. Hill, and C. C. Kak, "Relationship of Animal Protein-rich Diet to Kidney Stone Formation and Calcium Metabolism," *Journal of Clinical Endocrinology and Metabolism* 66 (1988): 140–46.

10. M. L. Brandi, "Flavenoids: Biochemical Effects on Therapeutic Applications," *Bone and Mineral* 19 (Suppl.) (1992): S3–S14.

11. E. Barret-Connor, J. C. Chang, S. L. Edelson, "Coffee-Associated Osteoporosis Offset by Daily Milk Consumption," *Journal of the American Medical Association* 271 (1994): 280–83.

12. T. L. Holbrook, "A Prospective Study of Alcohol Consumption and Bone Mineral Density," *British Medical Journal* 306 (1993): 1506–09.

13. Morris Notelovitz, M.D., and Diana Tonnessen, *Menopause and Midlife Health* (New York: St. Martin's Press, 1993), 102.

14. M. A. Fiatarone, E. Marks, N. Ryan, et al., "High Intensity Strength Training in Nonagenarians," *Journal of the American Medical Association* 263 (1990): 3029–34.

15. John F. Aloia, M.D., et al., "Prevention of Involutional Bone Loss by Exercise," *Annals of Internal Medicine* 89 (1978): 356–58.

16. Richard Prince, Margaret Smith, Ian Dick, et al., "Prevention of Premenopausal Osteoporosis," *New England Journal of Medicine* 325 (1991): 1189.

17. Barbara S. Hulka, M.D., Lloyd E. Chambles, Ph.D., David Kaufman, M.D., et al., "Protection Against Endometrial Carcinoma by Combination-Product Oral Contraceptives," *Journal of the American Medical Association* 247 (1982): 475–77.

18. J. Hargrove, W. Maxson, A. Wentz, and L. Burnett, "Menopausal Hormone Replacement Therapy with Continuous Daily Oral Micronized Estradiol and Progesterone," *Obstetrics and Gynecology* 73 (1989): 606.

19. John Lee, M.D., *Natural Progesterone: The Multiple Roles of a Remarkable Hormone*, (Sebastopol CA: BLL Publishing, 1993), 54.

20. John Lee, M.D., "Osteoporosis Reversal with Transdermal Progesterone," *Lancet* 336 (1990): 1327.

21. V. Matkovic and R. Heaney, "Calcium Balance During Human Growth Evidence for Threshold Behavior," *American Journal of Clinical Nutrition* 55 (1992): 992–96.

22. B. J. Abelow, T. R. Holford, and K. L. Insogna, "Cross-Cultural Association Between Dietary Animal Protein and Hip Fracture: A Hypothesis," *Calcif Tissue* 50 (1992): 1448.

23. D. W. Dempster and R. Lindsay, "Pathogenesis of Osteoporosis," *Lancet* 341 (1993): 797–805.

24. Robert Recker, M.D., "Calcium Absorption and Achlorhydria," *New England Journal of Medicine* 313 (1985): 70.

25. Susan Whiting, "Safety of Some Calcium Supplements Questioned," *Nutrition Reviews* 52 (1994): 95–97.

26. R. W. Smith, W. R. Eyler, and R. C. Mellinger, "On the Incidence of Senile Osteoporosis," *Annals of Internal Medicine* 52 (1960): 773–76.

27. M. Chapuy, M. Arlot, F. Duboeuf, et al., "Vitamin D-3 and Calcium to Prevent Hip Fractures in Elderly Women," *New England Journal of Medicine* 327 (1992): 1637–1642.

28. L. Bitensky, J. Hart, A. Catterall, et al., "Circulating Vitamin K Levels in Patients with Fractures," *Journal of Bone and Joint Surgery* 70-B (1988): 663–64.

29. F. H. Nielson, C. D. Hunt, L. M. Mullen, and J. R. Hunt, "Effect of Dietary Boron on Mineral, Estrogen, and Testosterone Metabolism in Postmenopausal Women," *FASEB Journal* 1 (1987): 394–97.

Chapter 8

1. M. L. Taymor, S. H. Sturgis, and C. Yahia, "The Etiological Role of Chronic Iron Deficiency in Production of Menorrhagia," *Journal of the American Medical Association* 187 (1964): 323–327.

2. M. S. Biskind and G. R. Biskind, "Effects of Vitamin B Complex Deficiency on Inactivated Estrone in the Liver," *Endocrinology* 31 (1942): 109.

3. H. L. Newbold, *Mega-Nutrients for Your Nerves* (New York: Berkley Publishing Co., 1975), 213.

4. Katharina Dalton, M.D., *Once a Month* (Alameda CA: Hunter House, 1994), 18.

5. Richard Passwater, *Evening Primrose Oil* (New Canaan CT: Keats Publishing, 1981), 22.

6. Kunin, *Mega-Nutrition for Women*, 76.

7. J. Minton, W. Foecking, et al. "Response of Fibrocystic Breast Disease to Caffeine Withdrawal and Correlation of Cyclic Nucleotides with Breast Disease," *American Journal of Obstetrics and Gynecology* 135 (1979): 157.

8. Penny Wise Budoff, M.D., *No More Menstrual Cramps and Other Good News* (New York: G. P. Putnam, 1981), 73.

9. P. M. Farrell and J. G. Bieri, "Megavitamin E Supplementation in Man," *American Journal of Clinical Nutrition* 28 (1975): 1381.

10. M. S. Biskind, "Nutritional Deficiency in the Etiology of Menorrhagia, Cystic Mastitis and Premenstrual Tension, Treatment with Vitamin B Complex," *Journal of Clinical Endocrinology and Metabolism* 3 (1943): 227.

11. R. A. Anderson, M. Polansky, N. Bryden, et al., "Urinary Chromium Excretion of Human Subjects: Effects of Chromium Supplementation and Glucose Loading," *American Journal of Clinical Nutrition* 36 (1982): 1184–93.

12. P. D. Leathwood and F. Chauffard, "Aqueous Extract of Valerian Reduces Latency to Fall Asleep in Man," *Planta Medica* (1985): 144–48.

13. M. X. Sullivan and W. C. Hess, "Cystein Content of Finger Nails in Arthritis," *Journal of Bone and Joint Surgery* 16 (1935): 185–88.

14. J. M. Kraemer, A. V. Michalek, L. Lininger, et al., "Effects of Manipulation of Dietary Fatty Acids on Clinical Manifestations of Rheumatoid Arthritis," *Lancet* 1 (1985): 184–187.

15. Norman Childers, *A Diet to Stop Arthritis* (Somerville NJ: Somerset Press, 1991).

16. L. G. Darlington, N. W. Ramsey, and J. C. Mansfield, "Placebo-Controlled, Blind Study of Dietary Manipulation Therapy in Rheumatoid Arthritis," *Lancet* (Feb. 1, 1986): 236.

17. E. R. Schwartz, "The Modulation of Osteoarthritis Development by Vitamin C and E," *International Journal of Vitamin and Nutrition Research* 26 (suppl.) (1984): 141–46.

18. I. Machtey and L. Ouaknine, "Tocopherol in Osteoarthritis: A Controlled Pilot Study," *Journal of the American Geriatric Society* 26 (1978): 328–30.

19. E. C. Barton-Wright and W. A. Elliot, "The Pantothenic Acid Metabolism of Rheumatoid Arthritis," *Lancet* 2 (1963): 862–63.

20. J. C. Arnand, "Osteoarthritis and Pantothenic Acid," *Lancet* 2 (1963): 1168.

21. Peter Simpkin, "Oral Zinc Sulphate in Rheumatoid Arthritis," *Lancet* ii (1976): 539.

22. Antoniohopes Vaz, "Double-Blind Clinical Evaluation of the Related Efficacy of Ibuprofen and Glucosamine Sulfate in the Management of the Knee In-Out Patients," *Current Medical Research and Opinion* 8 (1982): 145–149.

23. P. M. Brooks, S. R. Potter, W. W. Buchanan, "NSAID and Osteoar-thritis—Help or Hindrance," *Journal of Rheumatology* 9 (1982): 3–5.

Chapter 9

1. Marianne Legato, M.D. and Carol Colman, *The Female Heart: The Truth About Women and Coronary Artery Disease* (New York: Simon and Schuster, 1992), xii.

2. Margie Patlak, "Women and Heart Disease," *FDA Consumer* 28 No. 9 (Nov. 1994): 7–10.

3. Legato, *The Female Heart*, 16.
4. T. Bush, L. Cowan, E. Barret-Connor, et al., "Estrogen Use and All-Cause Mortality," *Journal of the American Medical Association* 249 (1983): 903–906.
5. Meir Stampfer and Graham Coldidz, "Estrogen Replacement Theory and Coronary Heart Disease: A Quantative Assessment of the Epidemiologic Evidence," *Preventive Medicine* 20 (1993): 47–63.
6. Erkki Hirvonon et al., "Effects of Different Progestogens on Lipoproteins During Postmenopausal Replacement Therapy," *New England Journal of Medicine* 304 (1981): 560–563.
7. K. Ten, H. Boman, and S. P. Darger, "Increased Frequency of Coronary Heart Disease in Relatives of Wives of Myocardial Infarct Survivors: Assortive Mating for Lifestyle and Risk Factors," *American Journal of Cardiology* 53 (1984): 399–403.
8. Marian Sandmaker, *The Healthy Heart Handbook* (National Institutes of Health Pub. No. 92–2720: 1992), 11.
9. Richard Helfant, M.D., *Women Take Heart* (New York: G.P. Putnam's Sons, 1993), 18.
10. Morris Notelovitz, M.D., and Diana Tonnessen, *Menopause and Midlife Health* (New York: St. Martin's Press, 1993), 327.
11. Helfant, *Women Take Heart*, 17.
12. Lewis Perdue, *The French Paradox and Beyond* (Sonoma CA: Renaissance Publications, 1992), 3.
13. E. N. Frankel, J. Kanner, J. B. German, et al., "Inhibition of Oxidation of Human Low-Density Lipoprotein by Phenolic Substances in Red Wine," *Lancet* 341 (1993): 454–57.
14. Elizabeth Barret-Connor et al., "Why Is Diabetes Mellitus a Stronger Risk Factor for Ischemic Heart Disease in Women?" *Journal of the American Medical Association* 265 (1991): 627–31.
15. J. E. Manson, G. A. Colditz, M. J. Stampfer, et al., "A Prospective Study of Obesity and Risk in Coronary Heart Disease in Women," *New England Journal of Medicine* 322 (1990): 882–89.
16. K. E. Powell, P. D. Thompson, I. J. Caspersen, and J. S. Kendrick, "Physical Activity and the Incidence of Coronary Heart Disease," *Annual Review of Public Health* 8 (1987): 253–287.
17. S. N. Blair, H. W. Kohl, R. S. Passengarger, et al., "Physical Fitness and All-Cause Mortality: A Prospective Study of Healthy Men and Women," *Journal of the American Medical Association* 262 (1987): 2395–2401.
18. J. S. House, K. R. Landis, and D. Umberson, "Social Relationships and Health," *Science* 241 (1988): 540–45.
19. L. Schervitz, L. E. Graham, G. Grandits, and J. Billings, "Speech Characteristics and Behavior-Type Assessment in the Multiple Risk Factor Intervention Trial (MRFIT)," *Journal of Behavioral Medicine* 10 (2) (1987): 173–95.

20. National Heart and Lung Institute, "What Every Woman Should Know About High Blook Pressure".

21. Boston Women's Health Book Collective, *The New Our Bodies, Ourselves* (New York: Simon and Schuster, 1984), 541.

22. R. Stamler et al., "Nutrition Therapy for High Blood Pressure: Final Report of a Four-Year Randomized Controlled Trial—The Hypertension Control Program," *Journal of the American Medical Association* 257 (March 20, 1987): 1484.

23. Herbert Benson, M.D., *The Mind/Body Effect: How Behavioral Medicine Can Show You the Way to Better Health* (New York: Berkley Books, 1981), 98.

24. Peter Wilson, "High-Density Lipoprotein, Low-Density Lipoprotein and Coronary Artery Disease," *The American Journal of Cardiology* 66 (1990): 7A–10A.

25. *Arteriol Thrombosis* 12 (1992): 529.

26. Bruce Kinosian, Henry Glick, and Gonzalo Garland, "Cholesterol and Coronary Heart Disease Predicting Risks by Levels and Ratios," *Annals of Internal Medicine*," 121 (1994): 641–47.

27. D. Ornish, S. Brown, L. Scherwitz, et al., "Can Lifestyle Changes Reverse Coronary Heart Disease?" *Lancet* 336 (1990): 129–33.

28. W. Willet, M. Stampfer, J. Manson, et al., "Intake of Trans Fatty Acids and Risk of Coronary Heart Disease Among Women," *Lancet* 341 (1193): 581–85.

29. W. Willet, et al., *Lancet*, 581–85.

30. D. Kromhout, E. Bosschieter, and C. Coulander, "The Inverse Relation Between Fish Consumption and 20-Year Mortality from Coronary Heart Disease," *The New England Journal of Medicine* 312 (1985): 1205–09.

31. Clemens Von Schacky, "Prophylaxis of Atherosclerosis with Marine Omega-3 Fatty Acids," *Annals of Internal Medicine* 107 (1987): 890–99.

32. Cynthia Ripson, Joseph Keenan, and David Jacobs, et al., "Oat Products and Lipid Lowering: A Meta-Analysis," *Journal of the American Medical Association* 267 (1992): 3317–25.

33. D. Hunninghake, V. Miller, J. LaRosa, et al., "Hypocholesterolemic Effects of a Dietary Fiber Supplement," *American Journal of Clinical Nutrition* 59 (1994): 1050–1054.

34. J. J. Cerda, F. L. Robbins, C. W. Burgin, et al., "The Effects of Grapefruit Pectin on Patients at Risk for Coronary Heart Disease Without Altering Diet or Lifestyle," *Clinical Cardiology* 11 (1988): 589–94.

35. T. Wolever, D. Jenkins, S. Mueller, et al., "Method of Administration Influences the Serum Cholesterol-Lowering Effect of Psyllium," *American Journal of Clinical Nutrition* 59 (1994): 1055–59.

36. D. Kritchevsky and C. Sirtori et al., *Nutrition in Cardio-Cerebrovascular Diseases* (March 15, 1993): 180–214.

37. M. Stampfer, C. Hennekens, J. Manson et al., "Vitamin E Consump-

tion and the Risk of Coronary Disease in Women," *The New England Journal of Medicine* 328 (1993): 1444–49.

38. J. Jandak and S. Richardson, "Alpha-Tocopherol, and Effective Inhibition of Platelet Adhesion," *Blood* 72 (1989): 141–49.

39. J. Hallfrisch, V. Singh, D. Muller et al., "High Plasma Vitamin C Associated with High Plasma HDL- and HDL-2 Cholesterol," *American Journal of Clinical Nutrition* 60 (1994): 100–5.

40. A. Kardinaal, F. Kok, J. Ringstad et al., "Antioxidants in Adipose Tissue and Risk of Myocardial Infarction: the EURAMIC Study," *Lancet* (1993): 1379–84.

41. JoAnn Munson, M.D., presented to American Heart Assocation, Anaheim CA, 1991.

42. Susan Peterson, "Beta Carotene, Vitamin E Cut Women's Heart Risk," *The Orange County Register* (November 14, 1991), 26.

43. Lars Brattstrom, Bjorn Hultberg, and Jan Erik Hardebo, "Folic Acid Responsive Postmenopausal Homocysteinemia," *Metabolism* 34 (1985): 107–77.

44. Meir Stampfer and Walter Willet, "Homocysteine and Marginal Vitamin D Deficiency: The Importance of Adequate Vitamin Intake," *Journal of the American Medical Association* 270 (1993): 2726–27.

45. E. Barrett-Connor, K. Khaw, and S. Yen, "A Prospective Study of Dehydroepiandrosterone Sulfate, Mortality, and Cardiovascular Disease," *The New England Journal of Medicine* 315 (1986): 1519–24.

46. L. E. Mitchell et al., "Evidence for an Association between Dehydroepiandosterone Sulfate and Nonfatal, Premature, Myocardial Infarction in Males," *Circulation* 89 (1994): 889–93.

47. Julian Whitaker, "DHEA Can Prevent Heart Disease," *Health and Healing* Vol 4 No 12 (1994): 7.

Chapter 10

1. Mortimer Zuckerman, ed., "Battling Breast Cancer," *U.S. News and World Report* (Nov. 23, 1992).

2. K. Steinberg, S. Thacker, J. Smith et al., "A Meta-Analysis of the Effect of Estrogen Replacement Therapy on the Risk of Breast Cancer," *Journal of the American Medical Association* 265 (1991): 1985–90.

3. "Hormones and Women's Health: Choices, Risks, and Benefits," newsletter (Washington DC: National Women's Health Network, 1993).

4. Morris Notelovitz, M.D., and Diana Tonnessen, *Menopause and Midlife Health* (New York: St. Martin's Press, 1993), 380.

5. A. H. Follingstad, "Estriol, the Forgotten Estrogen?" *Journal of the American Medical Association* 239 (1978): 29–30.

6. Ronald Watson and Tina Leonard, "Selenium and Vitamins A, E, and C. Nutrients with Cancer Prevention Properties," *Journal of the American Dietetic Association* 86 (1986): 505.

7. Henry Dreher, *Your Defense Against Cancer* (New York: Harper and

Row, 1988), 8.

8. U.S. Department of Health and Human Services, *Diet, Nutrition, and Cancer Prevention: The Good News* (NIH Pub. 87–2878). (Washington DC: Government Printing Office, 1987).

9. Kenneth Carroll, "Dietary Fats and Cancer," *American Journal of Clinical Nutrition* 53 (1991): 1064S–1067S.

10. L. A. Cohen, D. P. Rose, and E. L. Wyndner, "A Rationale for Dietary Intervention in Postmenopausal Breast Cancer Patients: An Update," *Nutritional Cancer* 19 (1993): 1–10.

11. H. P. Lee, L. Gourley, S. W. Duffy, et al., "Dietary Effects on Breast Cancer Risk in Singapore." *Lancet* 337 (1991): 1197–1200.

12. A. P. Simpoulos, "Summary of the NATO Advanced Research Workshop on Dietary Omega-3 and Omega-6 Fatty Acids: Biologic Effects and Nutritional Essentials," *Journal of Nutritional Medicine* 119 (1989): 521–28.

13. Julie Corliss, "Seafood Fatty Acids May Lower Cancer Risk," *Journal of the National Cancer Institute* 81 (1989): 1530–31.

14. L. A. Cohen, M. E. Kendall, E. Zang, C. Meschter, and D. P. Rose, "Modulation of N-Nitrosomethylurea-Induced Mammary L-Tumor Promotion by Dietary Fiber and Fat," *Journal of National Cancer Institute* 83 (1991): 496–501.

15. Nicholas Petrakis and Eileen King, "Cytological Abnormalities in Nipple Asperates of Breast Fluid from Women with Severe Constipation," *Lancet* (November 28, 1981): 1204.

16. J. L. Marx, "Oxygen Free Radicals Linked to Many Diseases," *Science* 235 (1987): 529–31.

17. W. J. Blot, Jun-Yao Li, P. R. Taylor et al., "Nutrition Intervention Trials in Linxian, China: Supplementation with Specific Vitamin/Mineral Combinations, Cancer Incidence, and Disease-Specific Mortality in the General Population," *Journal of the National Cancer Institute* 85 (1993): 1483–92.

18. D. Hunter, J. Manson, G. Colditz et al., "A Prospective Study of the Intake of Vitamins C, E, and A and the Risk of Breast Cancer," *New England Journal of Medicine* 329 (1993): 234–40.

19. Ibid.

20. H. Stahelin, K. Gey, and E. Ludin, "Beta Carotene and Cancer Prevention: The Basel Study," *American Journal of Clinical Nutrition* 53 (1991): 265S–9S.

21. K. F. Gey, G. B. Brubacher, and H. B. Stahelin, "Plasma Levels of Antioxidant Vitamins in Relation to Ischemic Heart Disease and Cancer, *American Journal of Clinical Nutrition* 45 (1987): 1368–77.

22. Glady Block, "Vitamin C and Cancer Prevention: The Epidemiologic Evidence," *American Journal of Clinical Nutrition* 53 (1991): 270S–282S.

23. S. G. Jenkinson, "Oxygen Toxicity," *Journal of Intensive Care Medicine* 3 (1988): 137–52.

24. P. Knekt, A. Aromaa, J. Maatela et al., "Vitamin E and Cancer Prevention," *American Journal of Clinical Nutrition* 53 (1991): 283S–286S.

25. N. J. Walt et al., *British Journal of Cancer Research* 49 (1984): 321.

26. Jeffrey Bland, "Safety Issues Regarding Supplements," Preventive Medicine Update Vol 13 No 3 (March 1993): 211.

27. J. Salonen, Jukka, Riitta Salonen et al., "Risk of Cancer and Vitamin A and E: Matched Case-Control Analysis of Prospective Data," *British Medical Journal* 290 (1985): 417.

28. G. N. Schraucer et al., *Japanese Journal of Cancer Research* 76 (May 1985): 374.

29. Larry C. Clark and Gerald Combs, "Selenium Compounds and the Prevention of Cancer: Research Needs and Public Health Implications," *Journal of Nutrition* 116 (1986): 170.

30. H. P. Lee, L. Gourley, S. W. Duffy et al., "Dietary Effects on Breast-Cancer Risk in Singapore," *Lancet* 337 (1991): 1197–200.

31. Mark Messina and Stephan Barnes, "Commentary: The Role of Soy Products in Reducing Risk of Cancer." *Journal of the National Cancer Institute* 83 (1991): 541–46.

32. *Journal of the National Cancer Institute* (1994).

Chapter 11

1. Jane Fonda with Mignon McCarthy, *Women Coming of Age* (New York: Simon and Schuster, 1984), 60.

2. Morris Notelovitz, M.D., and Diana Tonnessen, *Menopause and Midlife Health* (New York: St. Martin's Press, 1993), 158.

3. Emrika Padus, *The Woman's Encyclopedia of Health and Natural Healing* (Emmaus PA: Rodale Press, 1981) 271.

4. Richard A. Kunin, M.D., *Mega-Nutrition for Women* (New York: McGraw-Hill, 1983), 46.

Chapter 12

1. R. Kuczmarski, K. Flegal, S. Campbell, and C. Johnson, "Increasing Prevalence of Overweight Among U.S. Adults," *Journal of the American Medical Association* 272 (1994): 205–11.

2. Cheraskin and Ringdorf, *Psychodietetics*, 30.

3. Jane Brody, "Research Suggests Pulling the Strings on Yo Yo Dieting," *The New York Times* (June 27, 1991).

4. Barbara Edelstein, M.D., *The Woman Doctor's Medical Guide for Women* (New York: William Morrow, 1982), 146.

5. W. Insull, M. Henderson, D. Thompson et al., "Results of a Randomized Feasibility Study of a Low-Fat Diet," *Archives of Internal Medicine* 150 (1990): 421–27.

6. S. Kayman, W. Bruvold, J. Stern, "Maintenance and Relapse After Weight Loss in Women: Behavioral Aspects," *American Journal of Clinical Nutrition* 52 (1990): 88–807.

Chapter 13

1. Sharie Miller, "Getting Started, Staying Fit," *Vogue* 175 (April 1985): 340.
2. Philip Elmer-Dewitt, "Extra Years for Extra Effort," *Time* (March 17, 1986): 66.
3. Richard A. Kunin, M.D., *Mega-Nutrition for Women* (New York: McGraw-Hill, 1983), 150.
4. Morris Notelovitz, M.D., and Diana Tonnessen, *Menopause and Midlife Health* (New York: St. Martin's Press, 1993), 329.
5. Kenneth H. Cooper, M.D., *The New Aerobics* (New York: Bantam Books, 1981), 16.
6. Covert Bailey, *Smart Exercises: Burning the Fat, Getting Fit* (Boston: Houghton Mifflin Company, 1994), 42.
7. Covert Bailey, *The Fit or Fat Woman* (Boston: Houghton Mifflin Company, 1989), 28.
8. J. F. Aloia, D. M. McGowan, A. N. Vaswani et al., "Relationship of Menopause to Skeletal Muscular Mass," *American Journal of Clinical Nutrition* 53 (1991):1378–83.
9. Notelovitz and Tonnessen, *Menopause and Midlife Health*, 102.
10. Bob Anderson, *Stretching* (Bolinas CA: Shelter Publications, 1980).

Chapter 14

1. Henry Beiler, *Food Is Your Best Medicine* (New York: Random House, 1965), 34.
2. U.S. Department of Health and Human Services, *Ten Leading Causes of Death in the U.S., 1977* (Washington DC: Government Printing Office, 1980).
3. Select Committee on Nutrition and Human Needs, U.S. Senate, *Dietary Goals for the United States* (Washington DC: Government Printing Office, 1977).
4. *Journal of the American Dietetic Association* (Sept. 1994).
5. Gladys Block, "Dietary Guidelines: The Results of Food Consumption Surveys," *American Journal of Clinical Nutrition* 53 (1991) 356S–357S.
6. *Benefits of Nutritional Supplementation*, Council for Responsible Nutrition (Washington DC: 1990).
7. R. S. Murphy and G. A. Muhad, "Methodologic Considerations of the National Health and Nutrition Examination Survey," *American Journal of Clinical Nutrition* (Suppl.) 35 (May 1982).
8. Ibid.
9. Sherwood L. Gorbach, M.D., David R. Zimmerman, and Margo Woods, *The Doctor's Anti-Breast Cancer Diet* (New York: Simon and Schuster, 1984), 15.
10. Weston Price, *Nutrition and Physical Degeneration* (Santa Monica CA: Price-Potter Foundation, 1970).

11. Richard A. Kunin, M.D., *Mega-Nutrition for Women* (New York: McGraw-Hill, 1983), 12.

Chapter 15

1. National Research Council, "Diet and Health Implications for Reducing Chronic Disease Risk," (Washington DC: National Academy Press, 1980).
2. Walter Willet, "Diet and Health: What Should We Eat?" *Science* 264 (1994): 532–37.

Chapter 16

1. "Pesticides in 61 Percent of Fruits, Vegetables," *Associated Press* (April 1994).
2. M. S. Biskind, "Nutritional Deficiencies in the Etiology of Menorrhagia, Cystic Mastitis and Premenstrual Tension, Treatment with Vitamin B Complex," *Journal of Clinical Endocrinology and Metabolism* 3 (1943): 227.
3. Lauersen and Stukane, *Listen to Your Body*, 120.
4. Peter W. Curatolo, M.D., and David Robertson, M.D., "The Health Consequences of Caffeine," *Annals of Internal Medicine* 98 (1983): 641–53.
5. Lynn Rosenberg et al., "Breast Cancer and Alcoholic Beverage Consumption," *Lancet* (January 30, 1982): 267–69.
6. Jeffrey Bland, Ph.D., *Nutraerobics*, (New York: Harper and Row, 1983), 214.

Chapter 17

1. Jeffrey Bland, Ph.D., *Nutraerobics* (New York: Harper and Row, 1983), 68.
2. *American Journal of Clinical Nutrition* 24 (1971): 269.

Chapter 18

1. Patricia Hausman, *The Right Dose: How to Take Vitamins and Minerals Safely* (Emmaus PA: Rodale Press, 1987).
2. Sheldon Saul Hendler, M.D., *The Doctors' Vitamin and Mineral Encyclopedia* (New York: Simon and Schuster, 1990), 428.

Glossary

Adipose (fat)—commonly used in describing the part of the body where fat is stored.

Adrenal glands—small, pyramid-shaped glands situated on top of each kidney that secrete various substances, among which are the steroid hormones androgen, estrogen, and progestogen.

Adrenal cortex—outer part of the adrenal gland that secretes cortisone-like hormones.

Adrenaline—neurotransmitter produced by the adrenal gland, released in response to fear, heightened emotion, or physiological stress.

Amenorrhea—failure to menstruate.

Amino acid—organic compound of carbon, hydrogen, oxygen, and nitrogen; the "building blocks" of protein.

Amphetamine—drug used as a stimulant for people in tired or depressed states; also used to decrease nasal congestion and to decrease appetite.

Androstenedione—weak androgen abundantly secreted by menopausal ovaries as well as the adrenal glands; a major source of estrogen during and after menopause.

Anovulatory cycle—menstrual cycle without ovulation or the release of an egg.

Antihypertensive—medication used to lower high blood pressure.

Antioxidant—substance that prevents oxidation or inhibits reactions promoted by oxygen.

Arteriosclerosis—a group of diseases characterized by thickening and loss of elasticity of artery walls; may be due to an accumulation of fibrous tissue, fatty substances, or minerals.

Atherosclerosis—a type of arteriosclerosis in which the inner layer of the artery wall is made thick and irregular by deposits of the fatty substance plaque.

Atrophy—withering of an organ that had previously been normally developed.

Basal metabolic rate (BMR)—temperature of the body at the time of awakening each morning.

Beta carotene—compound in plants that the body converts into vitamin A.

Bioflavenoid—constituent of the vitamin C complex.

Blood-sugar control mechanism—regulates the amount of sugar in the blood-stream; includes the pancreas, insulin, glucagen, and adrenaline.

Blood-sugar level—amount of glucose (sugar) circulating in the blood-stream (normal levels are between 80 and 120 milligrams).

Calcitonin—"calcium sparing" hormone released primarily by the thyroid gland; acts to slow down the breakdown of bone.

Calcium balance—net processes in which calcium enters the body (through the diet) and leaves the body (through sweat, urine, and feces).

Carotid arteries—large arteries on either side of the neck that supply blood to the head.

Catecholamines—breakdown products of adrenaline.

Cellulose—carbohydrate found in the woody part of plants and trees; pro-vides fiber to the body.

Cervix—narrow lower end of the uterus that extends into the vagina.

Chelation—process of covering a mineral with an amino acid to enhance its absorption rate.

Cholesterol—a fatlike substance found in the cell walls of all animals, including humans; some cholesterol is manufactured in the body and some comes from foods of animal origin that we eat.

Collagen—protein that is the supportive component of bone, connective tissue, cartilage, and skin.

Corpus luteum—"yellow body" seen in the ovary after ovulation, the cells of which produce progesterone, estrogen, and other hormones.

Corticosteroids—drugs that resemble the adrenal hormones.

Cortisone—adrenal hormone that can be harmful to bones; also a drug that resembles the adrenal hormone.

Cysteine—sulfur-containing amino acid.

Deoxyribonucleic acid (DNA)—the fundamental component of living mat-ter.

Diuretic—agent that promotes the excretion of urine.

Dopamine—important brain neurotransmitter that plays a role in body movement, motivation, primitive drives, sexual behavior, emotions, and immune system function.

Double-blind study—study in which neither the experimenter nor the sub-jects know who is getting what treatment.

Dysmenorrhea—painful or difficult menstruation.

Edema—excessive accumulation of fluid in tissues, causing swelling.

Endocrine glands—glands that manufacture hormones and release them into the bloodstream (such as adrenal glands, ovaries, and pancreas).

Endorphins—natural opiatelike substances in the brain that control pain, among other things.

Enzyme—protein capable of producing or accelerating a specific biochemical reaction at body temperature.

Epidemiological study—study of the occurrence and prevalence of disease.

Estrogen—class of female sex hormones found in both men and women, but in larger proportions in women; primarily responsible for the development and maintenance of female sex characteristics and reproductive functions in women.

Estrone—weaker form of estrogen.

Fibroids—fibrous, noncancerous growths most commonly found in or on the uterus.

Follicle—small, round sac; in the ovary, each egg is contained in a follicle.

Follicle-stimulating hormone (FSH)—hormone secreted by the pituitary gland that stimulates the follicles in the ovary to grow and mature.

Free radicals—highly reactive molecular fragments, generally harmful to the body.

Gammalinolenic acid (GLA)—polyunsaturated fat used by the body to produce certain prostaglandins that control several important body processes.

Glucose—simple sugar that is the usual form in which the carbohydrate exists in the bloodstream.

Glucose tolerance factor (GTF)—a chromium compound that aids insulin in the control of blood sugar.

Glycogen—principal form in which a carbohydrate is stored in the body for ready conversion into energy; found in the liver and muscle tissue in particular.

Hemoglobin—protein in the blood that contains iron and carries oxygen from the lungs to the tissues.

High density lipoprotein (HDL)—the smallest lipoprotein, which removes cholesterol from LDL and cells and transports it back to the liver, where cholesterol is broken down into bile acids and excreted into the intestine; high levels are associated with low risk of heart disease.

Histamine—compound found in many tissues that is responsible for the increased permeability of blood vessels and plays a major role in allergic reactions.

Homeostasis—body's tendency to maintain a steady state of equilibrium despite external changes.

Hormone—chemical substance produced in one part of the body and carried in the blood to another part of the body, where it has specific effects.

Hydrogenation—addition of hydrogen to any unsaturated compound (oils are changed to solid fats by this process).

Hypoglycemia—low or falling concentration of glucose in the bloodstream, often caused by an excessive intake of refined carbohydrates in the diet.

Hypothalamus—part of the brain containing groups of nerve cells that control temperature, sleep, water balance, and other chemical and visceral activities.

Hysterectomy—surgical removal of the uterus (a radical hysterectomy includes removal of the uterus, cervix, ovaries, egg tubes, and sometimes lymph nodes near the ovaries).

Incontinence—inability to control urine retention.

Insulin—protein hormone secreted by the pancreas into the blood; regulates carbohydrate, fat, and protein metabolism.

Labia majora—major lips or folds of skin of the female external genitals, located on either side of the entrance to the vagina.

Lactase—intestinal enzyme that breaks down lactose (a sugar) into easily digested compounds.

Lactobacillus acidophilus—class of "friendly" bacteria found in yogurt and other milk products; also found in both the intestines and the vagina, where it controls the growth of yeast.

Lactose—sugar found in milk and other dairy products.

Lactose intolerance—deficiency of the lactase enzyme, which results in uncomfortable gastrointestinal symptoms when foods containing lactose are eaten.

Lecithin—waxlike substance with emulsifying and antioxidant properties, found in animals and plants.

Lipoprotein—a complex particle consisting of lipid (fat), protein, and cholesterol molecules bound together to transport fat through the blood.

Low-density lipoprotein (LDL)—particles that are rich in cholesterol; high levels in the blood are associated with the premature development of atherosclerosis and an increased risk of heart disease.

Luteinizing hormone (LH)—hormone produced by the pituitary (a large surge of this hormone in each menstrual cycle precedes ovulation by 12 to 24 hours).

Menarche—beginning of menstruation.

Menorrhagia—excessive bleeding during menstruation.

Metabolism—sum of chemical changes; the building up or destruction of cells that takes place in the body.

Monounsaturated fat—a fat chemically constituted to be capable of absorbing additional hydrogen; these fats have been shown to lower blood cholesterol levels (olive oil, for example).

Neurotransmitter—substance that transmits nerve impulses across a synapse; brain chemicals that are involved in carrying messages to and from the brain.

Oophorectomy—removal of the ovaries (also called ovariectomy).

Osteopenia—lower than normal bone mass.

Ovary—one of two female organs containing the eggs and the cells that produce the female hormones estrogen and progesterone.

Ovulation—process during which a mature egg is released from the ovary.

Oxalates—compounds that can interfere with the absorption of calcium; found in some leafy green vegetables, such as spinach.

Oxidation—process of combining with oxygen.

Pancreas—large glandular organ, extending across the upper abdomen close to the liver, that secretes digestive juices into the intestinal tract; it contains enzymes that act upon protein, fat, and carbohydrates; also secretes the hormone insulin directly into the blood.

Phytates—phosphorus-containing compounds that can interfere with the absorption of calcium; found in the outer husk of cereal grains.

Phytohormones—plant substances that are structurally and functionally similar to human steroids; they exert a very weak effect on the body.

Pituitary gland—small, oval organ at the base of the brain that produces many important hormones (particularly FSH and LH) and has been called "the master gland."

Placebo—pill having no medicinal value, often used as a control in an experimental situation.

Plaque—a deposit of fatty (and other) substances in the inner lining of the artery wall, characteristic of atherosclerosis.

Platelets—substances in the blood that help form blood clots.

Progesterone—hormone produced by the ovary during the second half of the menstrual cycle; promotes the growth of the uterine lining prior to menstruation and, in pregnancy, the growth of the placenta.

Progestins—synthetic version of the female hormone progesterone.

Progestogens—group of synthetic steroid hormones that include progesterone and other hormones that have similar effects.

Prostaglandins—one of several compounds formed from essential fatty acids and whose activities affect the nervous, circulatory, and reproductive systems and metabolism; research indicates that a type of prostaglandin is implicated in muscular contractions and menstrual cramps.

Ribonucleic acid (RNA)—compound of nucleic acid responsible for the transmission of inherited traits.

Serotonin—substance present in many tissues (especially the blood and nerve tissue) that stimulates a variety of smooth muscles and nerves and is believed to function as a neurotransmitter.

Syndrome—set of symptoms that occur together.

Testosterone—strongest of the male sex hormones, found in both women and men but in much greater proportions in men.

Thyroid gland—organ at the base of the neck primarily responsible for regulating the rate of metabolism.

Tinctures—powdered herbs that are added to a 50-50 solution of alcohol and water.

Triglyceride—the main type of lipid (fatty substance) found in the fat tissue of the body and also the main type of fat found in food; high levels in the blood are associated with a greater risk of coronary atherosclerosis.

Uterus—complex female organ composed of smooth muscle and glandular lining; the womb.

Vagina—muscular canal in the female that extends from the vulva to the cervix.

Vasodilation—enlargement or dilation of blood vessels.

Vulva—external female sex organ, composed of the major and minor lips (labia majora and minora), the clitoris, and the opening of the vagina.

Resources

BOOKS

Beauty

Vera Brown, with Patricia Culligan, *Vera Brown's Natural Beauty Book* (Mountain View CA: Anderson World Books, 1981).

Diet

Benjamin T. Burton, *The Heinz Handbook of Nutrition* (New York: McGraw-Hill, 1976).

Robert Haas, Ph.D., *Eat to Succeed* (New York: Onyx Books, 1986).

Marin Katahn, Ph.D., *The 200 Calorie Solution* (New York: Berkley Books, 1982).

Susie Orbach, *Fat Is a Feminist Issue* (New York: Berkley Books, 1978).

Debra Waterhouse, *Outsmarting the Female Fat Cell* (New York: Hyperion, 1993).

Exercise

Bob Anderson, *Stretching* (Bolinas CA: Shelter Publications, 1980).

Sheila Cluff with Eve Shaw, *Sheila Cluff's Aerobic Body Contouring: The New Low-Impact Exercise Program for the Ageless Body* (Emmaus PA: Rodale Press, 1987).

Covert Bailey, *Fit or Fat* (Boston: Houghton Mifflin, 1977).

Covert Bailey and Lea Bishop, *The Fit or Fat Woman* (Boston: Houghton Mifflin Company, 1989).

Kenneth Cooper, M.D., *The New Aerobics* (New York: Bantam Books, 1970).

Jane Fonda with Mignon McCarthy, *Women Coming of Age* (New York: Simon and Schuster, 1984).

Richard Hittleman, *Richard Hittleman's Yoga: 28-Day Exercise Plan*, (New York: Bantam Books, 1969).

General Information and Interest

Boston Women's Health Book Collective, *The New Our Bodies, Ourselves* (New York: Simon and Schuster, 1984).

Paula B. Doress-Worters and Diana Laskin Siegal, *The New Ourselves, Growing Older* (New York: Simon and Schuster, 1994).

Jennifer Louden, *The Woman's Comfort Book: A Self-Nurturing Guide for Restoring Balance in Your Life* (San Francisco: Harper San Francisco, 1992).

Anne Morrow Lindbergh, *Gift from the Sea* (New York: Pantheon, 1955).

Kaylan Pickford, *Always a Woman* (New York: Bantam Books, 1982).

Alexandra Stoddard, *Living a Beautiful Life: 500 Ways to Add Elegance, Order, Beauty and Joy to Every Day of Your Life* (New York: Avon Books, 1986).

Andrew Weil, *Health and Healing* (Boston: Houghton Mifflin, 1983).

Heart Health

Neil Gordon, M.D., and Larry Gibbons, M.D., *The Cooper Clinic Cardiac Rehabilitation Program* (New York: Simon and Schuster, 1990).

Marianne J. Legato, M.D., and Carol Colman, *The Female Heart: The Truth About Women and Coronary Artery Disease* (New York: Simon and Schuster, 1992).

Dean Ornish, M.D., *Dr. Dean Ornish's Program for Reversing Heart Disease* (New York: Random House, 1990).

Hormones and Health

Sandra Coney, *The Menopause Industry: How the Medical Establishment Exploits Women* (Alameda CA: Hunter House, 1994).

Susan Lark, M.D., *The Estrogen Decision* (Los Altos CA: Westchester Publishing Company, 1994).

John Lee, M.D., *Natural Progesterone: The Multiple Roles of a Remarkable Hormone* (BLL Publishing, P.O. Box 2068, Sebastopol CA 95473), 1993.

Carol Ann Rinzler, *Estrogen and Breast Cancer: A Warning to Women*, (New York: Macmillan Publishing Company, 1993).

Midlife Health

Lonnie Barbach, Ph.D., *The Pause: Positive Approaches to Menopause* (New York: Penguin Books, 1994).

Alan R. Gaby, M.D., *Preventing and Reversing Osteoporosis* (Rocklin CA: Prima Publishing, 1994).

Morris Notelovitz, M.D., and Diana Tonnessen, *Menopause and Midlife Health* (New York: St. Martin's Press, 1993).

Midlife Issues

William Bridges, *Transitions: Making Sense of Life's Changes* (Reading MA: Addison-Wesley Publishing Company, 1980).

Allan B. Chinen, M.D., *Once upon a Midlife: Classic Stories and Mythic Tales to Illuminate the Middle Years* (New York: Jeremy P. Tarcher/Perigee, 1992).

Clarissa Pinkola Estes, Ph.D., *Women Who Run with the Wolves* (New York: Ballantine Books, 1992).

Sue Monk Kidd, *When the Heart Waits: Spiritual Direction for Life's Sacred Questions* (San Francisco: Harper San Francisco, 1990).

Dena Taylor and Amber Coverdale Sumrall, eds., *Women of the 14th Moon: Writings on Menopause*, (Freedom CA: The Crossing Press, 1991).

Judith Viorst, *Necessary Losses: The Loves, Illusions, Dependencies and Impossible Expectations That All of Us Have to Give Up in Order to Grow* (New York: Fawcett Gold Metal, 1986).

Nutrition

Jeffrey Bland, *Nutraerobics: Dr. Jeffrey Bland's Complete Individualized Nutrition and Fitness Program for Life After 30* (San Francisco: Harper and Row, 1983).

Mark Bricklin, *The Natural Healing Cookbook* (Emmaus PA: Rodale Press, 1981).

Patricia Housman, *The Right Dose: How to Take Vitamins and Minerals Safely* (Emmaus PA: Rodale Press, 1987).

F. M. Lappe, *Diet for a Small Planet: Tenth Anniversary Edition* (New York: Ballantine Books, 1982).

Mark Messina, Ph.D., Virginia Messina, with Ken Setchell, Ph.D., *The Simple Soybean and Your Health* (Garden City Park NY: Avery Publishing Group, 1994).

Laurel Robertson et al., *Laurel's Kitchen: A Handbook for Vegetarian Cookery and Nutrition* (Petaluma CA: Nilgiri Press, 1976).

Women's Health

Barbara Edelstein, M.D., *The Woman Doctor's Medical Guide for Women* (New York: William Morrow, 1982).

Federation of Feminist Women's Health Centers, *A New View of a Woman's Body* (New York: Simon and Schuster, 1981).

Niels Lauersen, M.D., and Eileen Stukane, *Listen to Your Body: A Gynecologist Answers Women's Most Intimate Questions* (New York: Berkley Books, 1982).

Linda Madaras, Jane Patterson, and Peter Schlick, *Womancare: A Gynecologic Guide to Your Body* (New York: Avon, 1981).

PAMPHLETS

"Menopause" (Washington DC: National Women's Health Network).

Robin Van Liew, "Herbal Remedies for Women" (New York: Feminist Health Works, 1980).

Maria Lopez, Judy Costlow, Edit Adams et al., *Menopause: A Self Care Manual* (Santa Fe NM: A Santa Fe Health Education Project).

NEWSLETTERS

Berkeley Wellness Newsletter
University of California, Berkeley
P.O. Box 10922
Des Moines IA 50340

Diet and Nutrition Letter
Tufts University
P.O. Box 2465
Boulder CO 80322

Hot Flash: Newsletter for Midlife and Older Women
Edited by Jane Porcino, Ph.D.
School of Allied Health
   Professionals
State University of New York
Stony Brook NY 11794

Midlife Wellness
Center for Climacteric Studies
University of Florida
901 NW 8th Avenue, Suite B1
Gainesville FL 32061

Women's Health Connection
P.O. Box 6338
Madison WI 53716-0338
(800) 366-6632

Women's Health Advocate Newsletter
P.O. Box 420235
Palm Coast FL 32142

MENOPAUSE CLINICS

Center for Climacteric Studies
University of Florida
901 NW 8th Avenue, Suite B1
Gainesville FL 32601

North American Menopause Society
University Hospitals Dept of OB/GYN
2074 Abington Road
Cleveland OH 44106

NATURAL HORMONES

Bajamar Women's Health Care (800) 255-8025

Women's International Pharmacy (800) 279-5708

Index

A

abdominal exercises, 294–30
abdominal pain, 71
acupuncture, 92
acidophilus, 72
acne, 180
acupuncture, 88
adaptogens, 39
adrenal glands, 25, 28, 50, 75, 76
adrenalin, 52
aerobic dance, 104
aflatoxins, 177
age at menopause, 12
aging, acceptance of, 14
agitation, 90
AIDS, 70
alcohol, 53, 62, 69, 73, 76, 77, 87, 103, 123, 177, 186, 254–256
alcohol and breast cancer, 145
alcohol and heart disease, 144–145
alcoholism, 53, 60
alfalfa, 44, 101
allergies, 76
allergies, food, 133–134
aluminum, 100
amenorrhea, 98; psychogenic, 20
amphetamines, 77
androgen, 32
androstenedione, 30
anemia, 47, 57–60, 90, 125
anorexia, 20, 98
anovulatory cycle, 27–28
antacids, 100
anti-inflammatory drugs, 136
antibiotics, 72
anticonvulsants, 99–100
antidepressants, 77
antihistamines, 69
antihypertensive drugs, 77, 149
antioxidants, 157–160
antioxidants and breast cancer, 171
anxiety, 51, 90
apartate, 59
apathy, 60, 90
arms, exercises, 286–293
arteriosclerosis, 141
arthritis, 131–137; supplements for, 137

arthritis and food allergies, 133–134
arthritis and nutrition, 131–137
ascorbate, 59
atherosclerosis, 141
athletes and osteoporosis, 98

B

backache, 74
bacteria, 71
barbiturates, 54
basal metabolic rate, 195
baths, 53, 88, 92, 120, 191
beta blockers, 54
beta carotene, 55, 118, 158, 159–160, 151
beta carotene and breast cancer, 171–172
beta-endorphins, 35
BHA, 158
BHT, 158
biofeedback, 53
bioflavenoids, 43–44, 69, 117–118, 132, 275; sources of, 44
biotin, 275
birth control pill, 128, 142, 148, 149, 151
birth control, 24
black cohosh, 101
bladder infections, 71–74
bleeding, heavy, 116
blood disorders, 224
blood histamine, 78
blood sugar, 39, 46, 47, 48–60, 127–129
blood sugar and insomnia, 127–128
blood sugar fluctuations, causes of, 129
blood sugar, low, 60; controlling, 54–57; diagnosing, 52; symptoms of, 49
body weight, low, and menopause, beginning of, 20
bone health and nutrients, 111–114
bone mineral density (BMD) tests, 95
bones (see also osteoporosis), 30, 32, 33, 93–114
borage, 44, 110, 114, 275; sources of 114, 275
Boston Women's Health Book Collective, 21